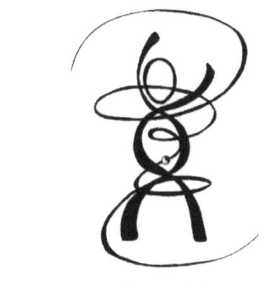

SPIRALING LIFE FORCE PRESS

Guiding Principles
of the Internal Arts

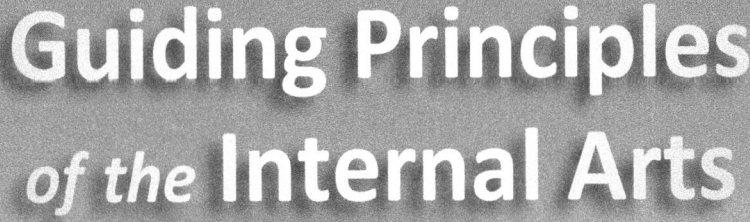

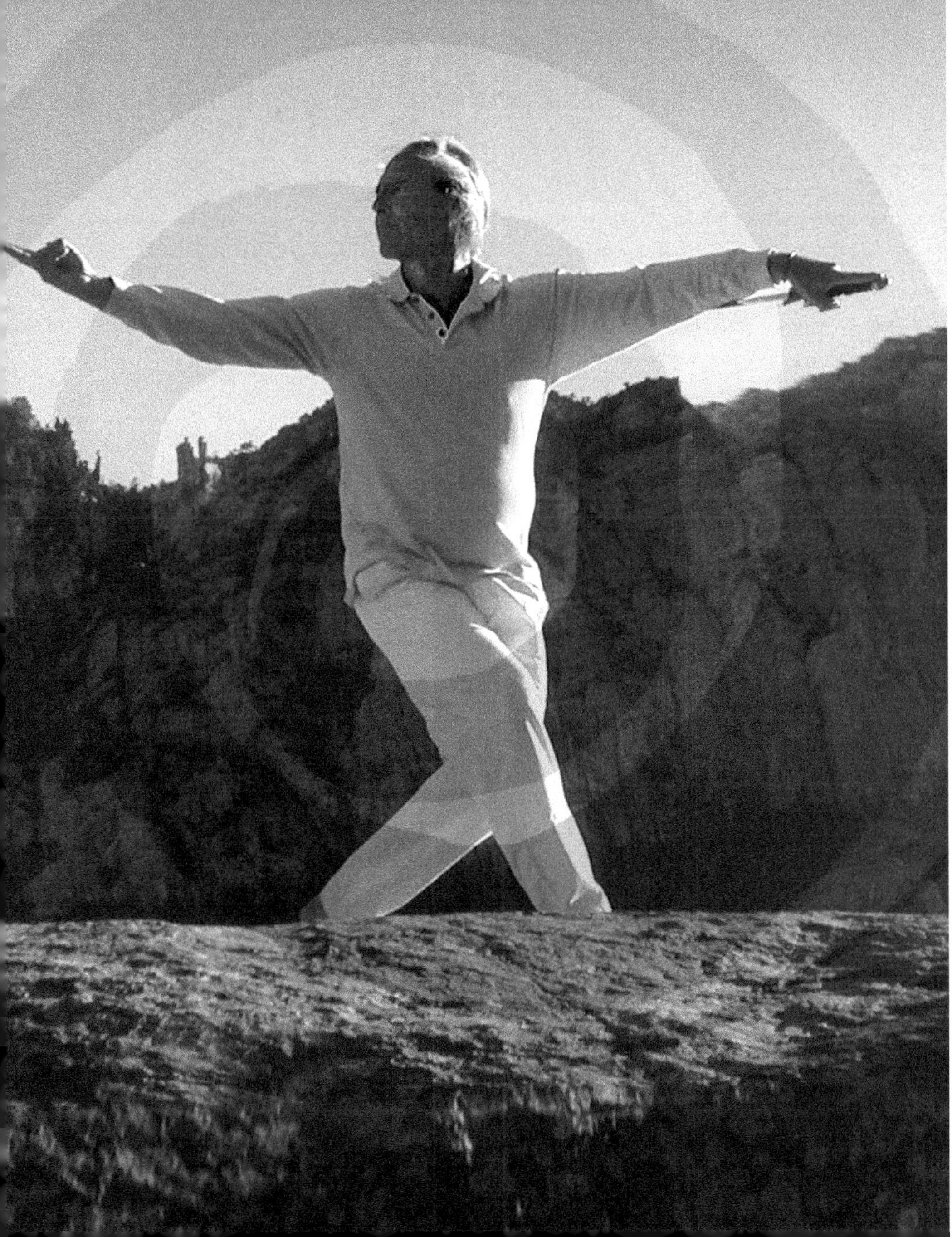

COPYRIGHT © 2013 BY LYN DILBECK
Guiding Principles of the Internal Arts
Cover Design: Peggy Sands, Indigo Disegno
Design, Photography, Illustration: Peggy Sands, Indigo Disegno
Back cover Photo: Peggy Sands, Indigo Disegno
Typesetting: Ingrid Hardy

No part of this book
may be used, reproduced or transmitted
in any form by any means, electronic or mechanical, including
photocopying and recording or by any information storage or retrieval
system, in any manner except in the case of brief quotations embodied
in critical articles and reviews. Request for such permission should be
submitted in writing to the author.
Spiraling Life Force • www.spiralinglifeforce.com

All rights reserved.
Printed in the United States of America.
First Edition September 30, 2013
ISBN: 978-0-9885414-0-5

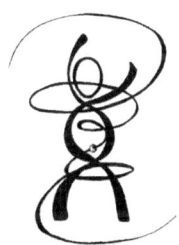

TABLE OF CONTENTS

I	**Introduction to the Manual and DVD**	3
	Theory	4
	From Theory to Practice, From Knowledge to Wisdom	6
	Balance and Integration	7
II	**Warming Up Your Body**	15
	Spinal Series ~ Enlivening the Five Pumps	16
	Vertical Stretch	16
	Slow Undulations with Forward and Back Hold	17
	Secret Thoracic Release	19
	Tan Tien Turning (the Spiral Pump)	20
	Push and Fall (the Side Pump)	22
	Single Knee Circles	24
III	**The Unity Form**	31
	• Opening	32
	1. Draw Earth Qi	32
	2. Cleaning the Rice (to the Right)	33
	3. Driving Qi Up the Midline, Elbows Leading	34
	4. Cleaning the Rice (to the Left)	35
	5. Driving Qi Up the Midline, Fingers Leading	35

TABLE OF CONTENTS cont.

    6. Drawing Heaven Qi 36
    7. Scooping Qi from Heaven (to the Right) 36
    8. Driving Qi Down the Midline, Fingers Leading 37
    9. Scooping Qi from Heaven (to the Left) 38
    10. Driving Qi Down the Midline, Elbows Leading 38
    11. Qi Comes Up the Rabbit Hole 39
    12. Repeat ~ Qi Comes Up the Rabbit Hole 40
    13. Qi Goes Down the Rabbit Hole 40
    14. Repeat ~ Qi Goes Down the Rabbit Hole 41
    15. Offering Your Heart 41
    16. Giving to the Kingdom, Receiving from the Kingdom 42
    17. The Heart Triangle 43
    18. Distributing and Balancing the Qi 44
    19. Prayer Hands 46
        • Close 47

IV The Guiding Principles 49
    1. Be in the Present Moment 50
    2. Stay Soft 53
    3. Allow the Yin and Yang to Form Their Union of Balance 55
        A. Rising/Expanding/Opening ~
            Sinking/Contracting/Closing 56
        B. Tension ~ Relaxation 57

TABLE OF CONTENTS cont.

    C. Origin of Yang ~ Origin of Yin 58
        • Chin Circling 58
    D. Releasing to Peng 59
    E. Outward Reaching ~ Inward Drawing 60
    F. Giving ~ Receiving 60
  4. Allow Your Body to Unify Physically and Energetically 60
    • Pushing the Wall, Pushing Another 61
    • Peng with a Partner 63
    • Contracting Peng 64
    • Silk Reeling Interconnection 60
  5. Express Greatly from Your Heart 66
  6. Use "Imaginitive Feeling" to Allow the Functions of
     Your Tan Tiens to Integrate 67
  7. What Happens in One Tan Tien, Happens in All Tan Tiens ... 70

V Causal Level of Qi Gong Practice 73
  Meditation of Three Levels 74
    • First Level 74
    • Second Level 77
    • Third Level 79

VI Astral Level of Qi Gong Practice 83
  About the Author 91

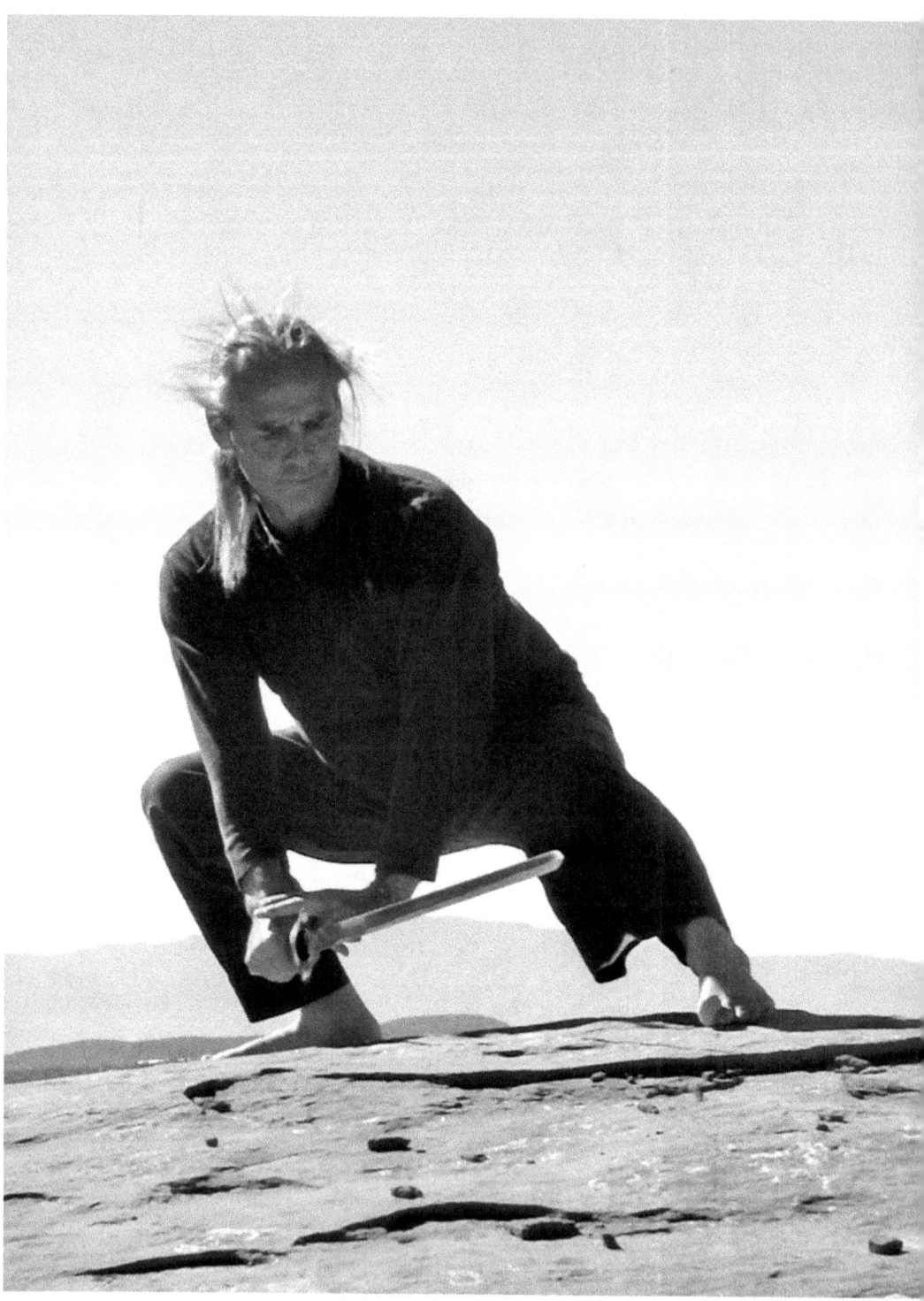

Authors Note

This life has been so full of learning experiences. Even at age 57, I am still learning.

The central theme in all of my lessons has been that absolutely everything I experience comes from me.... all of my experiences are reflections of the parts of my Soul (God within me) that I have chosen to hold in my consciousness as my truth. But the other central theme running right along with the first is that Who I Am does not come from any of my experiences. Now there's an oxymoron for you. Everything I experience comes from me, it is a reflection of me, but I do not come from any of my experiences. Wow, you could write a book on just that!

The beauty and the genius of the relationship between God and Creation, as it relates to us, is that both are always talking to us. God as our Soul is being reflected to our consciousness by Creation continually. They are guiding and helping us by showing us through our experiences what we are choosing to believe, and more specifically, who we are choosing to believe we are.

This gets even more interesting. Everything we experience as our reality is actually one of two things: it is either a reflection of who we believe we are (the beliefs we have chosen to hold in our consciousness), or it is a version of the opposite side of these beliefs. Our experiences of the opposite side of our beliefs are usually the reflections of our fears of not being, doing or having our beliefs. But it also works in reverse... our experiences can arise out of our desire to no longer be, do, or have what we are presently experiencing ~ our deeper desire to experience something "better." Our experiences of these latter reflections clearly demonstrate how our consciousness does evolve, how we do grow through all of our experiences, even the contracting or "bad" ones.

The power that brings the versions of the opposite sides of our beliefs into our reality arises from our attaching:
- The seeking of our identity and personal value in our experiences
- The attaching of our consciousness to the reflections in the Qi (Creation) of the beliefs we are choosing to hold onto.

This attachment manifests through our desire to be, do, or have something vibrational, something in this world, and through our fear of not being, doing, or having these same somethings.

The efficiency of this power to bring these opposite

versions of our beliefs into our reality is in direct proportion to the intensity or fervor of our attaching ~ how much we are seeking and trying to find our identity, value, purpose, and joy in our experiences. This intensity of our attaching becomes the intensity of our desires, which in turn becomes the intensity of our fears.

The more we hold onto any experience, the more apt we are to experience, again and again, its opposing side. The intensity of our desire to be, do, or have anything, and the intensity of our attempts to make it real, attracts the experience of not being, doing, or having it. This is because from our desire comes our fear, the fear of not being, doing, or having what we want. And when we fear anything a lot, we, in our attempting to not be, do, or have it, bring it into our reality. Through our fear actions, we can literally push away all the other possibilities of love and joy.

This is why we must remember Who We Are. We must remember that we do not come from what we are experiencing within Creation.

Relating to Another

This same dynamic of course occurs in our relationships with others.

We have chosen to hold the belief that we are not one with God, Creation, and our brothers and sisters. We also believe that we are not whole within ourselves and are limited in our power to manifest. We therefore experience within Creation the reflections of these beliefs and have attached to our experiences of needing and seeking something from another to find fulfillment – to become whole.

According to our unique beliefs about our own separation and what we believe we need, we experience the desire that love must show up in certain, specific ways. As shared above, these desires form our fears. Through the intensity of our attaching to the experiences of needing something from another, we can actually push that person away. Our fear of not having them and our fear of love not showing up in the specific ways we want it, or perceive we need it in order to feel complete and fulfilled, can blind us to the other expressions of love our partners can and want to give us. In our over attachment, we can "not see" all of the love that is there; we can literally "not see" all of the One we love.

I have learned these things because I have done all of them, many times.

Simple Truths

- Everything you experience comes from you... it is a reflection of your beliefs

- Nothing you experience is Who You Are

- What you experience is a reflection of what you are

choosing to believe, or it is a version of the opposite side of these beliefs.

- The manifesting power that brings into your reality the experiences of the opposite side of your beliefs is the intensity of how you, as consciousness, attach to your experiences (the fervor of your desiring and attempts [actions] to find your identity and personal value in your experiences).

The Key
Experience all things while remembering that you are the Consciousness of God, the Oneness and Love unifying God, Creation, and all life.

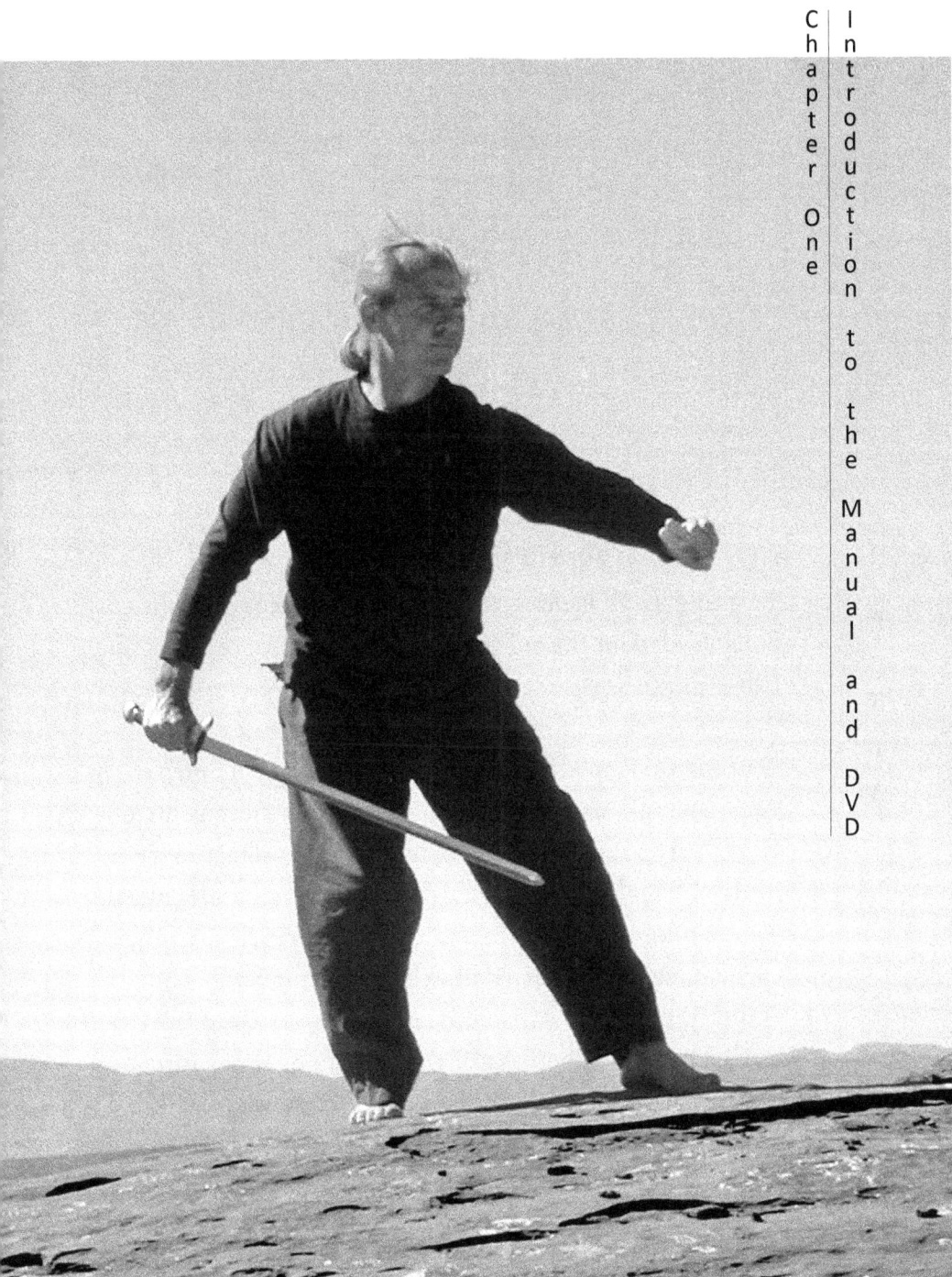

Chapter One | Introduction to the Manual and DVD

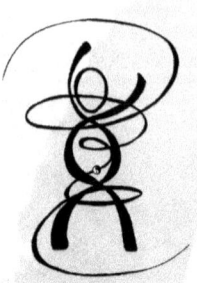

THE FIRST INSTRUCTIONAL MANUAL of this series, *"Starting Your Practice"*, helped you develop the physical skills needed for the energetic or etheric practice of Qi Gong. These skills were then codified in the *Foundation Form*.

This manual now presents the *Guiding Principles* of Qi Gong and will instruct you in how to apply these principles in the primary levels of existence: physical/energetic (Etheric), feeling/emotional (Astral), and mental (Causal). It is through the application of these principles to your experiences on all levels of existence that you realize the unbinding of your consciousness from the Qi of Creation and from the reflections of the beliefs of separation and limitation you have chosen to experience within Her.

Theory

In Qi Gong theory, there is only one thing. We have given

this one thing many names, but for the sake of brevity, lets call it God. Since there is only God, you are this one God. You are also God's extension as Creation, and you are God and Creation's ability to experience the apparent levels and facets of themselves/yourself. In your human form, these levels and facets are your Soul, consciousness, and mental-emotional-energetic-physical bodies.

In this understanding, you are the one source of all experiences. You do not come from nor are you defined by your thoughts, feelings, or perceptions of energy and matter. Also being God's consciousness, it is you that is choosing these experiences you are having. Your sense of being this oneness and your sense of responsibility to this oneness constitute the true, navigational star for the path of Qi Gong Practice.

We have all lost sight of this star. We have forgotten Who We Are. Our infinite consciousness has chosen to believe in a power that opposes God, opposes Oneness. Through this choice, we have identified with and therefore bound ourselves to the Qi that forms the vibrational planes of Creation, and we have bound ourselves to our experiences of being separate and limited.

Now experiencing yourself and your world as separate and limited, you have come to believe that you are lacking, that you must get something from Creation and your fellow beings to be whole and find value. Subsequently, you spend your time judging Creation according to your perceived needs, and then seek to control, manipulate, and own Her.

From Theory to Practice, From Knowledge to Wisdom

It is not by theory alone that you reawaken. You must walk the path that starts where you are now; you must turn this spiritual knowledge into a living wisdom.

As you enter onto the path of Qi Gong Practice, the navigational star dawns again in your consciousness. It is there, reminding you continually that your identity, value, and purpose come from God, not from Creation or from the experiences you are having within Creation. This knowledge then becomes your ability to release your perceived need to attach to Creation, and it becomes your courage to let go of your attachments to what you are experiencing within her. This releasing and letting go is the *Essence Movement* of Qi Gong. You are literally practicing how to experience vibrational existence while truly knowing that you do not come from these experiences.

The spiritual theory of Qi Gong becomes a method for living your life through the *Keys for the Transformation of Human Consciousness* (these four keys are presented and explained in the book **"Experiencing God's Reflection ~ The Role Qi Gong Plays in the Transformation of Consciousness."** They are Trust, Allowance, Surrender and <u>Non Attachment to Outcome</u>). But it is in your tan tiens, where these transformational keys are actualized or play out as the *Guiding Principles*, that the practice of Qi Gong takes place.

In your spiritual life, the Guiding Principles are where the rubber meets the road. These principles help you, as consciousness, relate to and interact with the Qi of energy, emotion, and thought. They show you how to experience all levels of Creation without judging controlling, and manipulating Her.

Balance and Integration

The purpose of the Guiding Principles is to allow two natural processes to occur ~ the process of balance and the process of integration. Balance and integration are the reflections, within the Qi, of the Love and Oneness of God and of your Soul.

It is you, through your perceived needs to judge, control, and manipulate the Qi and what you experience within the Qi, that is disrupting these processes. As you apply the Guiding Principles to your experiences, you stop interfering with the Qi's gong, Her natural processes. You continue to experience Creation, but you at the same time suspend judging, controlling, manipulating, and needing to own Her. You, in essence, allow Creation (God Your Mother) to form Her supreme balance, the balance in which you experience God and your Soul reflected perfectly. This is an important part of your letting go.

You cannot do this practice without trusting your Soul (God within you) and trusting the intelligence and forces of Creation (God Your Mother). This is an important way that the theory translates into the practice... you remember that your Soul is God, the one source of all experiences, and Creation is God Your Mother, the extension of God as the yin and yang forces of Qi and the divine intelligence orchestrating their balanced exchange (their giving and receiving of one another). Remember, it is in the balance between these forces of yin and yang that the reflections of God's Love and Oneness appear as your experiences.

More than trust, you must also have courage, for you and I have become so very attached to our experiences. In our coming to believe that our joy, well being, and even our existence depends on their outcome, we find it difficult to stop our habits of judging, controlling, manipulating and owning Creation.

Process of Balance

Every reflection of God in every realm of Creation... your thoughts within the Causal, your feelings and emotions within the Astral, and your perceptions of energy and matter within the Etheric... is experienced by you as having opposing sides, a yin side and a yang side. This is the divided nature or duality of your present world.

Every thought only has meaning in relativity to a complementary or comparative thought. Every feeling and emotion has two opposing sides. Every expression of energy is a sine wave (~) formed from peaks and troughs, and every atom is formed in opposing electro-magnetic charges (+ and -).

In the vibrational plane of energy and matter, the Etheric Plane, the two sides of your experiences show up as the following dualities:

Effort	Release
Doing	Non doing
Movement	Stillness
Tension	Relaxation
Expand	Contract
Open	Close
Rise	Sink
Move forward	Move back
Move right	Move left
Spiral right	Spiral left
Outside	Inside
Full	Empty

The dualities that form your experiences in the plane of feeling and emotion, the Astral Plane, are these:

Reaction	Repression
Desire	Fear
Attraction	Repulsion

Acceptance	Rejection
Giving	Receiving
Pleasure	Pain
Happiness	Sadness

And in the vibrational plane of thought, the Causal Plane, these are the dualities of your experiences:

I am this	I am that
Future	Past
Here	There
Believing	Not believing
Knowing	Not knowing
I do this	I don't do this (I do that)
I have this	I don't have this (I have that)
Success	Failure
Good	Bad
Right	Wrong

When you choose to attach your consciousness to the yang side of any experience, you make real the yin, and you will then also experience the yin side. And when you attach your consciousness to the yin, the yang becomes real to you, and you will then also experience the yang side.

Out of the untruth that there exists a power that opposes God arose yet another untruth that you and I have chosen to believe in: **we can achieve God or earn our way into the infinity and eternity of heaven by choosing to think,**

feel, be, or do what we experience as the right or good thing, and by not thinking, feeling, being, or doing what we perceive to be the wrong or bad thing. Hidden within this untruth are the beliefs that we must therefore judge our every experience, and we must control and manipulate them to our benefit. In our choice to hold on to these beliefs as our truth, and through each act we do in this life that is motivated by these beliefs, we not only cause the opposing sides of our experiences, but we are also binding our consciousness to the ongoing experiences of both.

The Guiding Principles are presented in chapter four. The first three principles:

- Be in the Present Moment
- Stay Soft
- Allow the Yin Qi and Yang Qi to Form Their Union of Balance,

focus on the process of balance. These principles of balance all share an essential formula ~ *allow the two sides of each experience, be it physical-energetic, feeling-emotional, or mental, to flow into one another.* Though this formula does not change throughout the practice of Qi Gong, you experience how it plays out differently depending on the vibrational plane in which you are having the experience. Always remember, it is the intelligence of Creation that you are trusting to orchestrate this marriage of opposites within you.

Integration

Integration is the other natural process that the Guiding Principles facilitate or focus on. When you apply these principles to your experiences, you are allowing Creation, by way of her natural laws of harmonics, to harmonize or reunite the apparent levels and parts of yourself and your reality... What happens within you happens without.

Expressed through the principles of integration are the sacred qualities of God's and also your Love. These qualities are the following:

<u>Absolute Inclusion</u> ~ you experience and accept every expression of life and aspect of Creation as part of yourself. You include everything and exclude nothing.

<u>Equality</u> ~ you experience the sanctity and equal importance of each part of Creation. You treat each life form and thing with reverence.

<u>Infinite Potential</u> ~ you see God's infinite potential in all things. You offer your help and guidance to every life form and piece of Creation in its evolution in consciousness.

As you study the Guiding Principles, you will see that the process of integration is emphasized in the 4th, 5th, 6th, and 7th principles and also in the meditation practice in chapter five.

Principle 4 — Allow Your Body to Energetically and
　　　　　　　Physically Unify

Principle 5 — Express Greatly from Your Heart

Principle 6 — Use "Imaginative Feeling" to Allow the
　　　　　　　Functions of Your Tan Tiens to Integrate

Principle 7 — What Happens in One Tan Tien Happens
　　　　　　　in all Tan Tiens

In the second level of the meditation practice (ch. 5), you are facilitating the integration of the vibrational levels of your being. In this part of the meditation, you allow your awareness to move freely through the Central Channel (the Chong Channel) of your body. Because this channel connects the three tan tiens together, you are, in a very direct way, reunifying yourself. Again remember, what happens within you happens without.

As you practice experiencing your life through all of the Guiding Principles, you will see that the natural processes of balance and integration overlap. When you are allowing balance to occur between the yin and yang forces of Qi on any level, you are, at the same time, facilitating both the reunification of the apparent pieces of yourself and Creation and the harmonization of the apparent levels within both of you.

Chapter Two | Warming Up Your Body

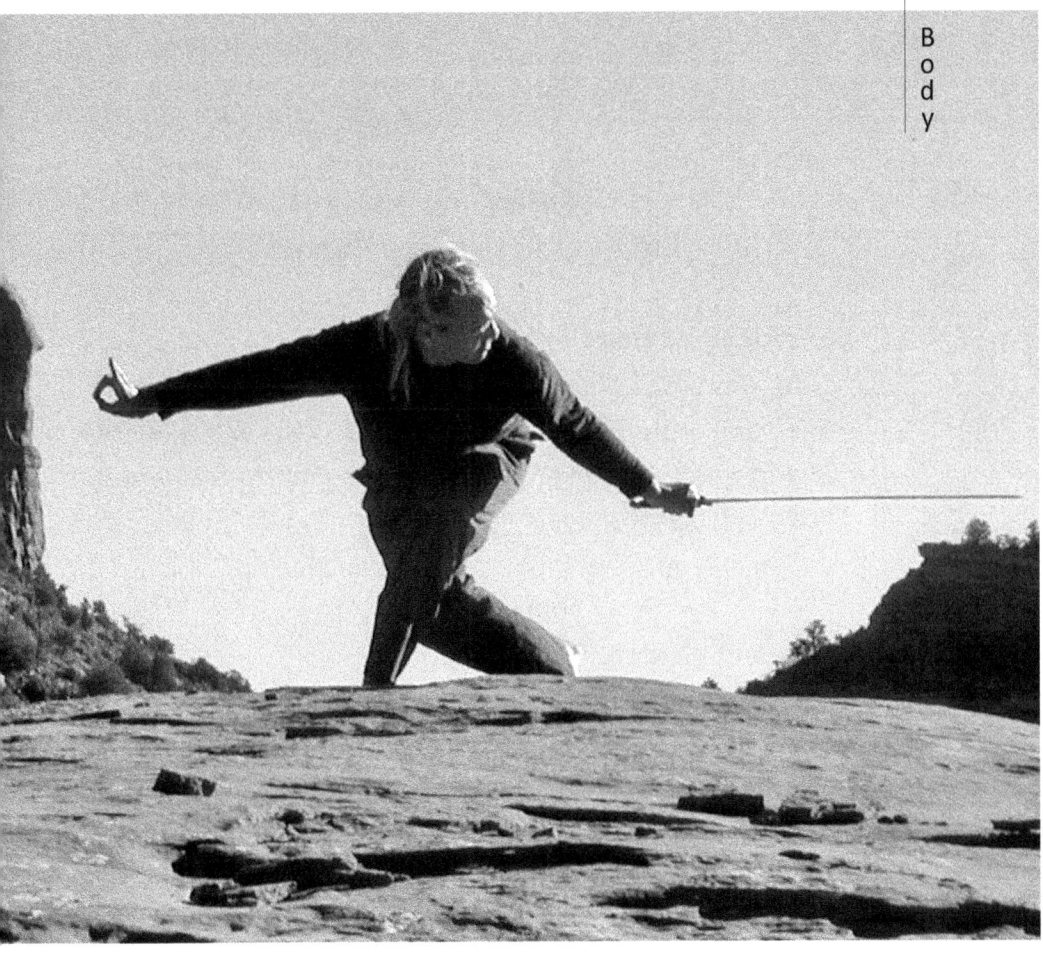

Spinal Series
Enlivening the Five Pumps

1. Vertical Stretch
- With your feet shoulder width apart, grab the back of one hand with the other (which hand grabs which is not important). Now extend your arms and hands above your head (palms facing up) and reach as high as you can continually for one minute, also be looking up. This feels like you are lifting yourself off the ground, though keep both feet planted.

- Then, as you continue to reach upward, bend your knees slightly to do the sink-fold-release. This release of your sacrum and tailbone will now create a downward, opposing pull, allowing a greater stretch of the lower back.

- Continue this stretch for another half minute, then drop

your arms and relax.

2. Slow Undulations with Forward and Back Hold

Slow Undulations

- Feet remain at shoulder width. Bend your knees and let your arms hang at your sides. Completely relax your spine, neck, and head so that your trunk and head slump forward.

- Your challenge here will be to maintain this deep, internal relaxation as you are moving your body forward and back.

- Initiate the forward movement in you shins. Stay relaxed as this movement then moves up through your knees, hips, spine, neck, and head like a wave. As each part sequentially moves forward, you will feel your relaxed neck and head starting to fall back.

- When your head is back, you must re-release... relax again your entire body from head to toe, before starting the back movement.

- Initiate the back movement in your calves. Stay relaxed as this movement moves up through your knees, hips, spine, neck, and head like a wave. As each part in turn is moving back, you will feel your relaxed neck and head falling forward.

- Undulate your body forward and back 9 times. Finish in the forward, slumped position.

Forward Hold
- Hold this forward, slumped position for 1 to 2 minutes. Keep your hips and pelvis in the sink-fold-release position, which places your dangling wrists at approximately knee height (the hips do not completely release which would place your hands close to the floor).

- Feel your complete, forward release that extends from the *Mingmen Point* (mid lumbar spine) up through your thoracic spine, neck, and head. Also feel your deep, opposing release, extending from the *Mingmen Point* down through your sacrum and tailbone.

- When you return to the standing position, be very careful to further bend your knees in order to gradually come out of this stretch.

Back Hold
- Move your feet apart to slightly wider than shoulder width, feet are parallel and your knees are bent. Bring your hands together at your forehead while interlacing your fingers.

- Now slowly release yourself back into a back bend. Keep your knees bent and allow the front of your body to open maximally. You are looking back and extending through the top of your head. Feel an energetic flow running through your spine... running through the arch formed from your legs, pelvis, spine, neck, and head.

- Hold this back release for as long as is comfortable for you. Shaking is a natural phenomenon, so do not fear it.

- When you are ready to return to the standing position, make sure to further bend your knees in order to ease yourself out of this deep stretch.

3. Secret Thoracic Release

- Bring your feet closer together, slightly less than shoulder width. For this release, you will keep your legs straight, so do not bend your knees but do not lock them either. Cross your arms in front of your chest while keeping your shoulders relaxed.

You are going to release the vertebrae in your thoracic spine (the rib part of your spine) by allowing them to lie over your inflated lungs. The feeling is similar to lying face down over one of those inflatable exercise balls. Your challenge will be to keep your spine, neck, and head, as well as your shoulders, completely relaxed as you are bending over your own, full lungs.

- Now take the deepest breath you can and hold it for as long as you can.

- While holding your breath, bend your body forward.

Remember, your legs remain straight. Your spine and shoulders are now completely relaxing onto your full lungs. Your crossed arms are dangling from your shoulders; your head, too, is just dangling.

- When you can hold your breath no longer, let it out and hang there for 20 to 30 seconds.

- Like in the other stretches, bend your knees to gently roll back up into the standing position.

- Good to repeat this release one more time.

4. Tan Tien Turning (the Spiral Pump)

- Move your feet back out to shoulder width or slightly wider, feet are parallel.

- Form your standing posture with its six adjustments: string, chin tuck, sink-fold-release, separated knees, knees bent, toes grab the earth; feel the heaviness of your relaxed internal organs pass down through your released low back, sacrum, and tailbone into your feet. At the same time feel your spine lengthening through the top of your head. The tip of your tongue touches the roof of your mouth. Release your arms and hands, allowing them to hang at your sides.

The challenge in this exercise, as I hope you remember from the first manual, is to allow the yin forces to match or stay in balance with the yang. In all of your movements, and especially so in the spiraling of your body, you must feel the heaviness of your internal organ release and the sustained softness within your sacral area (yin) as being equal (as a force) to your feeling of the active push from your legs and the active turning of the three tan tiens (yang). In other words, your release/sink must remain equal to your effort/rise.

Remember that in your physical body, your Lower Tan Tien manifests as your legs and pelvis, your Middle Tan Tien as your spine and chest, and the Upper Tan Tien as your neck and head.

- Lightly push from your right foot to turn your legs and pelvis (Lower Tan Tien) to the left. In the action of turning your legs and pelvis, you also are turning your spine and chest and your neck and head.

- After your Lower Tan Tien comes to its natural stop, proceed to turn your spine and chest to their natural stop.

- And finally, turn your neck and head even further to their stop.

- Then lightly push from your left foot to sequentially turn your three tan tiens to the right. When doing this movement slowly, there is little to no transfer of weight, little to no side-to-side movement of your body.

- After turning your tan tiens 5 or 6 times in each direction slowly, increase the power of your pushes and the speed of the turnings. Your completely relaxed arms will naturally swing out from your body. Do your best to not control your arms, instead develop and easy swing-right, swing-left rhythm.

- The stronger you push and faster you turn, the more the yang forces express in you. So really focus on allowing the yin forces to have their equal expression.

- Do the Tan Tien Turning for 1 to 2 minutes.

5. Push and Fall (the Side Pump)

This is the fifth and last of your internal pumps:

1. Hip-Knee Pump ⎫	naturally express as you sink
2. Spinal Pump ⎬	& rise and in the forward-back
3. Chest Pump ⎭	undulating
4. Spiral Pump	— expresses in Tan Tien Turning
5. Side Pump	— expresses in Push & Fall

- Bring your feet closer together, about 14 inches apart. Your feet are parallel. Keep your shoulders and arms completely relaxed; they simply dangle at your sides. Finally, do not turn your body in this movement, your pelvis and chest remain forward facing.

- Now push from your left foot and left big toe. This feels similar to the way a ballerina would push herself off the floor. At the end of this push, both legs are straight and only the big toe of your left foot is touching the earth. Your right foot remains planted. In this pushing, you will feel the energy of the push moving up through your spine to the top of your head.

- While sustaining this push and feeling of the rising energy, allow your spine, neck, and head to fall to the left; you are allowing your spine, neck, and head to relax onto the energy that is coming up through your body from your left foot.

- While in this position, there is a tendency to lean forward and drop your head forward, so please pay attention to the following two adjustments:

  — First, gently push your pelvis forward until you feel that the opening of your vertebrae and ribs is perfectly along your side, not anterior or posterior. You will also feel your chest opening and your scapulae releasing.

  — Second, without lifting your head, turn it slightly to gaze at the sky.

- In preparation to do the move on the other side, bend both knees in order to sink straight down (your left heel touches the earth) and return to center where you are weighted equally in both feet. At this point you are slightly crouched.

- Now push from your right foot and right big toe while simultaneously allowing your spine, neck, and head to fall to the right. Pay attention to the adjustment of your pelvis and the adjustment of your head.

- Then bend both knees to sink straight down and return to center.

- Do this movement as a continuous side-to-side dance for two minutes, allowing the yang (push) and yin (fall or release) forces to flow into one another.

- Finish by holding the push-fall movement for about a minute on each side.

The Spinal Series ~ Enlivening the Five Pumps ends here. I often use this series as my warm-up routine before I practice the forms. But the Spinal Series does not warm up your ankles, knees, and hips sufficiently.

Single Knee Circles

At this juncture, I am going to share an important movement that not only warms up the leg joints, but also forms the foundation or root of the peng force that feeds the other internal movements:

— The lengthening and shortening of the spine
— The opening and closing of the chest
— The spiral and counter spiraling within the legs, pelvis, and spine
— The flexion (bending) and extension (straightening) of the four limbs
— And the spiraling-counter spiraling within your arms and hands

Needless to say, mastering this exercise, knowing and being comfortable with this level of the peng force, is essential to the etheric practice of Qi Gong.

• Start with your feet together. Pivoting on the heel, turn your right foot out to just shy of 90°. Bend your right knee and put your weight into your right leg.

• Then step forward with your left approximately 2 feet, making sure that you have a 4-inch channel running between your feet from front to back. The toes of your left foot point straight forward. Bend both knees and distribute your weight equally into both legs. You are facing 45° to the right.

• Now turn your pelvis and chest to the left in order to place both hands on your left knee.

• You are now in a crouched position with your left thigh being almost parallel with the floor. It feels like you are sitting on a low stool. You are obviously bent at the cua (your pelvic crease) but not overly so, your trunk is pretty much upright with just a slight forward incline. Your low back, sacrum, and tailbone are, of course, released. There is a tendency here to bend too far forward which does not allow you to drop your internal organs, therefore loosing your internal down (your internal heaviness).

You are now going to use your peng force to move your left knee through a small circle. This requires that you allow the rising-expanding forces (yang) that naturally express up through you when you push against the earth to flow into the sinking-contracting forces (yin) that naturally express down through you when you relax. You must push and relax at the same time. This mixing of forces happens throughout your entire body and also fills the energetic field surrounding you.

The push comes primarily from your back leg. The relaxing is in your internal organs and your low back, sacrum, and tailbone. Your pushing leg is like a geyser shooting up out of the earth, and your relaxed internal organs and sacral area are like you (your body) sitting down on that geyser and opposing its forces with your natural heaviness. Where these forces come together makes quite a spray. It is this "spray" that drives your movements and, in this case, drives your knee through a small circle.

- Push from your back right foot, which will start to move your body forward. But as soon as you feel the push energy coming up through you, completely relax your internal organs. Allow their heaviness to pass down through you, to pass down through your released low back, sacrum, and tailbone, in order to flow into both legs (but primarily into your back, right leg).

- This is not so much a forward and back movement (though your body will move forward and back to some extent) as it is an expanding and contracting movement. When you push and release at the same time, you will experience an expanding in the ligament structure of your ankles, knees, and hips. This will drive your left knee through the first half, the outward moving half, of its circle. When you stop the push from your back right leg, the ligaments naturally contract, which will draw the knee back in through the return half of its circle.

- Though you are focusing on the circling of your front knee, you will experience the back knee expanding and contracting as well.

- Do nine circles with your left knee in one direction and then nine more in the other direction.

- Repeat this exercise on the other side. Start with your feet together, then pivot your left foot out to just shy of 90°. Bend your left knee, placing all your weight in your left leg. Now step forward with your right approximately 2 feet, making sure, again, that you have a 4-inch channel. The toes of your right foot point straight forward. Bend both knees, distributing your weight equally into both legs. You are facing 45° to the left. Then turn your pelvis and chest to the right in order to place both hands on your right knee.

30

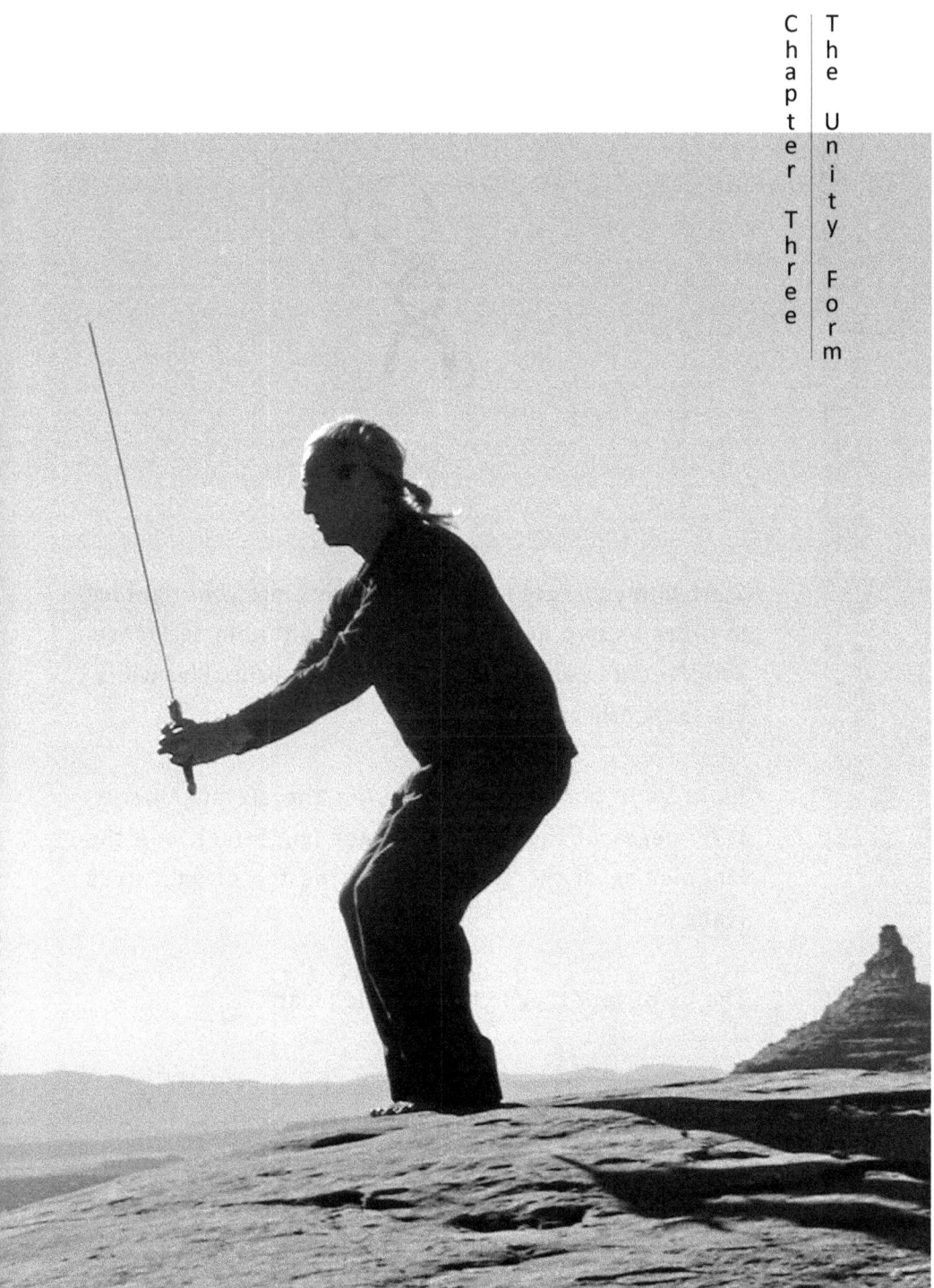

Chapter Three | The Unity Form

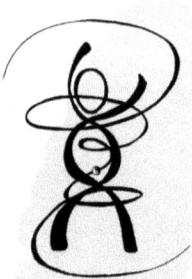

Opening

- Start with your feet together. Now sink into your right leg in order to step out with the left into the Horse Stance. Your feet are parallel, slightly wider than shoulder width, knees slightly bent.

- Build your posture remembering the six alignments, the release of the internal organs (yin force), and the lengthening of the spine through the top of your head (yang force).

- The tip of your tongue touches the palate.

1. Draw Earth Qi

- Extend both arms forward and approximately 30° to the sides. Your hands are just below belly button height with the palms facing down. Elbows are in front of your body, and slightly bent so that the tips of your elbows are pointing down (they are closer together than the wrists).

- Slightly flex your wrists so your palms face the earth. Keep your hands aligned with your forearms.

- Spread your fingers and thumbs in order to open the palms.

- Hold for one minute.

2. Cleaning The Rice (to the right)

- Initiating the movement by pushing from your left foot, turn your body to the right. Remember, this is a two-part turning: turn your legs and pelvis to their natural stop (Lower Tan Tien), then turn your spine and chest (Middle Tan Tien).

- Your left, extended arm moves to the right, hand staying below belly button height. Your open palm is facing the earth ~ like cleaning rice.

- Your right hand moves toward the belly button, palm facing the earth ~ like you are gathering something into the Lower Tan Tien.

- Now turn your body left, initiating the movement by pushing from your right foot (remember the two-part turning).

- The hands now change positions with the right arm extending to clean the rice, your left moves toward the belly button to gather into the Lower Tan Tien.

- After a few cycles, leave your right arm out in front as your body is turning left, and bring your left arm adjacent to the right arm, as your body is turning right.

- You are now facing forward with both arms extended forward. Hands are shoulder width apart at Lower Tan Tien height. Your open palms are facing the earth.

Breathing: Inhale on the Lower Tan Tien portion of the turns (legs and pelvis), exhale on the Middle Tan Tien portion of the turns (spine and chest).

3. Driving Qi Up the Midline, Elbows Leading

- Exhale: As you sink, lower both arms completely.

- Inhale: As you rise, both elbows come up the front of the body to their highest possible position above your head. The forearms, wrists, and hands remain relaxed.

- Then the forearms and hands engage to open up and out like the unfolding of a flower, palms are spread and face up, both arms come down through your sides to shoulder height.

- Exhale: While sinking slightly, lower your arms to waist height.

- Bring both arms out front, palms rotate to face down.

4. Cleaning the Rice (to the left)
- Initiating the movement by pushing from your right foot, turn your body to the left (remember the two-part turning).

- This time after a few cycles, leave your left arm out in front as your body is turning right, and bring your right arm adjacent to the left arm as the body is turning left.

- You are now facing forward with both arms extended forward. Hands are shoulder width apart at Lower Tan Tien height, open palms facing the earth.

5. Driving Qi Up the Midline, Fingers Leading
- Exhale: As you sink, both palms trace over the top, down the front, and along the bottom of the "Qi-Ball" (a field of energy in front of the lower abdomen and pelvis, approximately the size of a beach ball). Then sink a bit more while lowering both elbows. This additional sinking allows you to bring the backs of the hand together with your fingers pointing up.

- Inhale: As you rise, the hands are driven up the midline, fingers leading (like a rocket shooting up the spine through the top of your head).

- Above your head, both hands rotate so that the palms

face heaven; both arms are spiraling inward toward the midline.

6. Drawing Heaven Qi

- The upward extended arms and open palms continue to support heaven (this position is like hitting a volley ball with your palms and fingers). Your gaze, too, is up.

- At the same time, slightly sink in order to release your sacrum and tailbone into the earth.

- Hold for one minute, breathing naturally.

7. Scooping Qi from Heaven (to the right)

- Rise.

- Initiate this movement by turning your body to the right.

- Remember, this is a two-part turning: turn your legs and pelvis to their natural stop, then continue to turn your spine and chest.

- Your left arm and hand extend toward heaven in a spiraling-scooping fashion (the little finger side of your hand and forearm feel like the edge of a trowel or spatula, scooping from left to right).

- At the same time, lower your right, open hand along the

left side of your face, the palm rotating to face you (this gesture invites the Qi to enter your head). On the first part of your turn, the heel of the palm descends to your jaw line. On the second part of your turn, it continues down to the right, upper chest, palm facing up.

- As you now turn your body left, the arms and hands change positions.

- The right hand rises straight up with a relaxed hand, wrist, and elbow to become the upward-reaching, spiraling-scooping hand.

- Your left open hand is drawn down along the right side of your face, the palm rotating to face you.

- After a few cycles, leave the right arm extended above your head as your body is turning left, and then bring the left arm adjacent to your right arm as your body turns right.

- You are now facing forward with both arms extended above your head, palms facing one another.

Breathing: Inhale on the Lower Tan Tien portion of your turns (legs and pelvis); exhale on the Middle Tan Tien portion of your turns (spine and chest).

8. Driving Qi Down the Midline, Fingers Leading
- Exhale: Bring the backs of your fingers together as the

fingers point down toward your head.

- While sinking, drive your hands down the midline, fingers leading (like diving down through your own head, spine, and tailbone into the earth).

- Inhale: While rising, bring your extended arms up through your sides, palms rotating to face up.

- Finish with both arms extended above your head, palms facing one another.

9. Scooping Qi from Heaven (to the left)

- Initiate this movement by turning your body to the left. Remember, this is a two-part turning.

- After a few cycles, leave the left arm extended above your head, as your body is turning right. Then bring your right arm adjacent to the left arm, as your body turns left.

- You are now facing forward with both arms extended above your head.

- Rotate your arms and hands so that your palms face heaven (Draw Heaven Qi position). This time you need not sink.

10. Driving Qi Down the Midline, Elbows Leading

- Exhale: As you sink, lower both upward facing palms down

the midline of your body to mid-calf level. This is done with a continuous spiraling motion (like lowering two tea cups from heaven). Your elbows are leading this descent and approach one another briefly as they are passing the solar plexus. At the bottom, your fingers are pointing towards one another, palms facing up.

- Inhale, and then exhale. While rising, bring your extended arms up through your sides to waist height; both palms are facing the earth.

11. Qi Comes Up the Rabbit Hole

- Inhale: Bring both extended arms in front of your body, palms still facing earth, waist height.

- Exhale: As you sink, both palms trace over the top, down the front, and along the bottom of the "Qi-Ball". Then sink a bit more while lowering both elbows. This allows you to bring the backs of your hands together with the fingers pointing up.

- Inhale: As you rise, drive your hands up the midline, fingers leading, to the Heart Point (middle of your chest).

- Now open your heart space while rotating your arms and hands so that both palms face up.

- At this point, your elbows are touching each other in front of the solar plexus, and both up-turned palms are in front of your shoulders. Your fingers are pointing out to the sides.

- Through your continuous rise and heart space opening, drive your spiraling arms and hands out to the sides, fingers leading. Your palms remain upward facing, rising no more than a few inches above shoulder height.

- Exhale: With a slight sink, lower your arms to waist height.

12. Repeat ~ Qi Comes Up the Rabbit Hole
- Inhale: Bring the extended arms in front of your body, rotating the palms to face earth.

- At the end of the move after the spiraling arms extend out to the sides with up-turned palms, exhale. Then inhale as you raise both arms through your sides to extend above your head, palms facing one another.

13. Qi Goes Down the Rabbit Hole
- Exhale: The backs of your fingers touch as you point your fingers down toward the crown of your head.

- While sinking, drive the hands down the midline, fingers leading, to the Heart Point.

- As you continue to sink, rotate both arms and hands so the palms face up and the fingers point towards your armpits (tea cup move). You continue to sink while you are driving your hands through your armpits.

- At this point you have sunk all the way down, your upturned palms have just passed through your pits.

- Inhale: Now drive from your legs to rise. Direct the Qi through your spine to drive the arms and hands out to your sides with a continuous spiraling, fingers leading. The palms remain upward facing almost to the end of the extension when they then rotate 360° to finish palms up, slightly above shoulder height.

- Exhale.

14. Repeat ~ Qi Goes Down the Rabbit Hole

- Inhale: Raise both arms through your sides to extend above your head, palms facing one another.

- Exhale: The backs of your fingers touch as you point your fingers down toward the crown of your head.

- At the end of the move after your spiraling arms extend out to the sides, bring both of your palms together in front of the Heart Point (prayer hand position).

15. Offering Your Heart

- Inhale: Rotate your palms to face up, drop your elbows,

the sides of your little fingers are touching. By opening your heart, extend both upward facing palms straight forward.

- Continue opening your heart and continue extending your arms until both arms are out to your sides, just a few inches above shoulder height.

- Exhale: As you sink, drop your elbows and just allow both of your hands to "fall" back into the Heart Point, palms facing one another, fingers pointing up (prayer hand position).

- Repeat two more times.

16. Giving to the Kingdom, Receiving from the Kingdom

- Extend both arms forward, breast height, palms facing one another.

- Inhale: Initiating the movement by pushing from your left foot, turn your body to the right. This again, is a two-part turning: turn your legs and pelvis to their natural stop, then turn your spine and chest.

- The left arm remains in place as the right, extended arm moves right approximately 110° (barely passing behind you). Watch the right hand, the palm is open and vertical, staying at breast height.

- Exhale: Your left elbow now bends to bring the open, vertical palm to face the Heart Point.

- Inhale: Turn your body left (two-part turning).

- Your right arm remains in place, though it will follow somewhat with the turning of the body.

- Watch your left, open, vertical palm extend outward from the body to catch the natural arc of the turn. The hand stays at breast height as it moves to the left, 110° position (barely passing behind you).

- Exhale: Your right elbow now bends to bring the open, vertical palm to face the Heart Point.

- Do three complete cycles, finishing on the left (left, open palm extended left to the 110° position, right open palm hovering over the Heart Point).

17. The Heart Triangle

- Turn your body to face forward. Bring both extended arms in front of your body, breast height, palms facing one another.

- Draw both vertical, open palms half way in toward the chest. Both elbows move slightly out to the sides to form The Heart Triangle. Your Heart Point is in the center of this triangle.

- Remember to keep the wrists in line with your forearms; fingers and thumbs are spread to open your palms. Aim the center of each of your palms (Lou Gong points) at the Heart Point (center of the chest).

- With your "Imaginative Feeling" move through the three internal phases of this movement:
    1. Direct the Qi coming from the center of your palms into the Heart Point, filling the entire chest area with Qi.
    2. Through your internal awareness, soften your physical heart more than you have ever done before. Feel the Qi entering your heart.
    3. And finally, allow your relaxed and contented heart to beam outward into infinity.

18. Distributing and Balancing the Qi
<u>Right Side</u>
- Exhale: Initiate the movement by turning your body left and sinking slightly.

- With the fingers leading, your right palm traces the "Heart-Qi-Ball" down to the solar plexus to enter the triangle from below. At the same time, also with the fingers leading, your left palm traces the "Heart-Qi-Ball" up to the sternal notch to enter the triangle from above.

- Inhale: Then rise while turning your body right. This is a two-part turning: legs and pelvis, followed by the spine and chest.

- Your right hand shoots up the midline, fingers leading, to extend straight up (like coming out of the crown of your head). Spiral your arm so the palm is rotating to face away from you.

- Your left hand shoots down the midline, fingers leading, to extend straight down (like coming out of your tailbone). Spiral your arm so the palm is rotating to also face away from you.

- Exhale: Sinking slightly, now turn your body left.

- With the fingers leading, both extended arms follow a big circle. The right arm is coming down trough your right side to again enter the triangle from below (from the solar plexus). The left arm is coming up through your left side to enter the triangle from above (from the sternal notch).

- Repeat three more times.

- Exhale: On the last cycle after the right extends straight up and the left extends straight down, face forward without sinking. Bring both arms into the "airplane position"… both arms extended out to the sides, shoulder height, palms facing down.

- Reform The Heart Triangle.

<u>Left Side</u>
- Exhale: Initiate the movement by turning your body right

and sinking slightly.

- With the fingers leading, your left palm traces the "Heart-Qi-Ball" down to the solar plexus to enter the triangle from below. And with fingers leading, your right palm traces the "Heart-Qi-Ball" up to the sternal notch to enter the triangle from above.

- Inhale: Then rise while turning your body left.

- The left hand shoots up the midline, the right hand shoots down the midline.

- Repeat three more times.

- Exhale: On the last cycle, after the left extends up and the right extends down, face forward without sinking. Bring both arms into the "airplane position"… both arms extend out to the sides, shoulder height, palms facing down.

19. Prayer Hands

- Bring your palms together in front of the Heart Point to form Prayer Hands.

- Adjust your posture, release your shoulders and elbows, feel a slight pressure between the palms.

- Through this position, deeply feel the holiness of Who You Are!

Close

- In front of your Heart Point, rotate the palms to face up, fingers pointing forward. Drop your elbows.

- Extend your arms forward, sides of little fingers touching.

- Separate your arms to just wider than the shoulders.

- Rotate both arms so the palms now face forward, fingers pointing upward.

- Lower both arms and hands like leaves floating to the bottom of a pond.

- Draw your left foot in adjacent to the right.

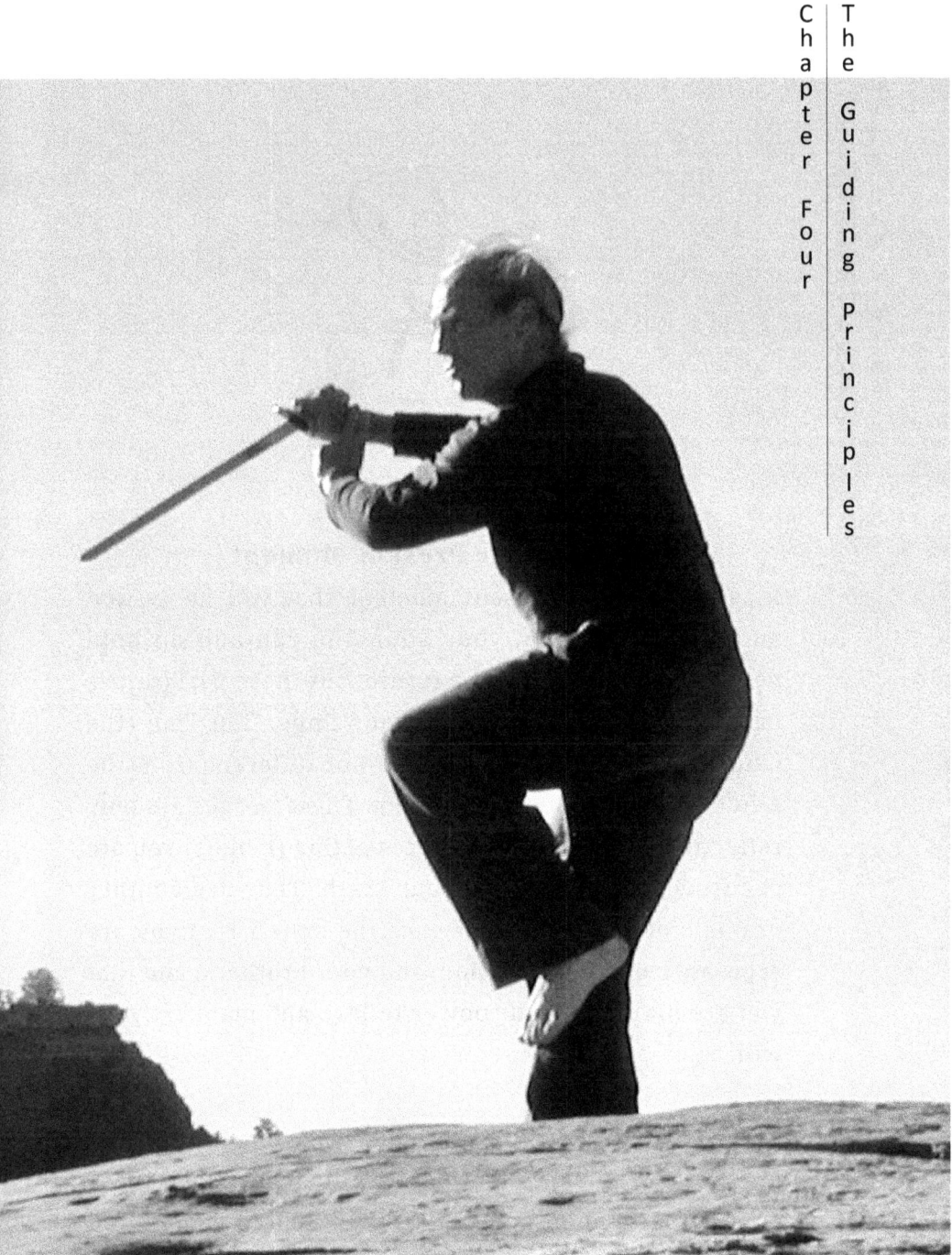

Chapter Four | The Guiding Principles

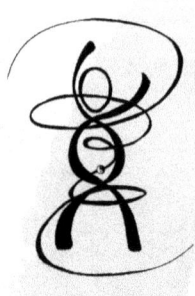

1. Be in the Present Moment

It is only in the present moment that you know God and God within you, your Soul. You can and do hold perceptions of a past and a future, but these past/future images you perceive through your Upper Tan Tien (the Causual Altar of you being) are not different from the other experiences you are having. These images are only reflections in the Qi of the pieces of God (beliefs) you are choosing to hold onto as your truth. They are another example of how you experience the beliefs that you are seperate from God, Creation, and your brothers; and that you are limited in your power to love and manifest your will.

Because you choose to experience fragments of God and not God's Wholeness or Oneness, does not make these perceptions true. It only makes them real to you. In God and in your Soul, you cannot be bound by time!

To be in the present moment does not mean that you are not aware of perceptions of a past and future. But in Qi Gong Practice you hold these images, or relate to them, in a "new way".... you experience them, but you do not attach to them; you do not seek your identity, value, or purpose in them.

In the present moment you can and do formulate plans and hopes. But as you hold these plans and hopes without attachment, you also do not overly concern yourself with how they will manifest or when they will manifest.... for you know that "the how" and "the when" are in the hands of the Qi (the intelligence and power of Creation). This is Her gong. With this trust and patience, your consciousness is freed to sense or "listen" to your Soul. You open yourself to receive soul guidance as to when to act and when to be still.

Even as you are aware of your perceptions of the past and future, you remember that your thoughts about the future are based in your perceptions of the past. Your future plans and hopes are a version of your past perceptions projected forward. As you experience these images without attaching and overly concerning yourself with them, you allow the Qi of your past and future thoughts to flow into one another. This forms a balance in the yin and yang Qi of your mind that permits you, as consciousness, to stay centered within the present.

Another characteristic of being in the present moment

is that you take your cues for how to live life from what appears before you. You live vulnerably without having to know all of life's outcomes. In this way you stop interfering in the natural balance of giving and receiving. You give more of yourself to life and do not restrict yourself in receiving what you have hoped for and everything else God and Creation want you to have. You open yourself to receive what you yet do not know. This is the path of true transformation by which you invite the Oneness and Love of God and Creation into your conscious experience.

Your ability and courage to live in this "new way" come out of your remembering Who You Are and out of the practice of implementing the *Transformational Keys* of <u>Trust</u>, <u>Allowance</u>, <u>Surrender</u>, and <u>Non-Attachment to Outcome</u>. These four keys are discussed in chapters 14-17 of "**Experiencing God's Reflection**".

This way of living in the present moment reminds me of an adage that says, "The real experiences of life are what happen to you on the way to your goal". It is in these "happenings" along the way that God and the Goddess (the intelligence and power of Creation) become apparent to us.

- Before warming up your body and practicing the form, take 2-3 minutes to allow your awareness, in every level of your being, to come into the present moment. This is an important part of **Entering the**

Qi Gong State (ch. 12 in the book, ch. 2 of Manual I).

- As you proceed with your practice of the form, remain consciously present in each moment of the form's unfolding. This is done by staying aware of and feeling the Guiding Principles of the practice as they are playing out through your body.

2. Stay Soft

Softness is the power of yin, the power to attract and draw. In you body (physical, emotional, and mental) softness acts much like a fluffy cotton ball that naturally wicks or absorbs. When you stay soft especially in and around your tan tiens, you draw the Qi of Creation into your energetic field. Your softness is your invitation to Her.

So you must have softness in your body while you are doing Qi Gong Practice. A great indicator of your body's overall softness and how well you are maintaining it is the area of your low back and sacrum. In Traditional Chinese Medicine this area is called Mingmen, the Gateway of Life. It is the back door to your Lower or Etheric Tan Tien, the field of intelligent power that governs your energetic/physical body. This area is hugely important for it is the meeting place of your spine, legs, and tailbone. It is the central point of intersection for the flow of yang Qi and therefore asks for its yin compliment. Your Mingmen asks for deep release!

The softness in the Mingmen area is the foundation of all

the yin (softness, relaxation, release, heaviness) in your body. Softness here translates into deeper relaxation in your tan tiens, in the joints of your arms (shoulders, elbows, wrists and hands), and in the joints of your legs (hips, knees, ankles, and feet). This softness not only facilitates the free movement of Qi through your trunk, neck, and head, but also allows your limbs to receive and be powered by these flows of Qi.

– When holding a posture or doing a movement, you must be conscious of keeping your low back, sacrum, and tailbone completely relaxed (soft).

– When engaging your arms, even when they are spiraling, you must keep them soft. This happens by "feeling" a heaviness in your shoulders, elbows and wrists.

– Allow all heaviness to pass down through your spine, sacrum, hips, knees, ankles, and feet as it is drawn to the center of the earth.

Four Continuous Bouncing
The most expedient way I know for developing, or finding again, the softness within your body and maintaining it, is to do Four Continuous Bouncing.

1. Bouncing in Standing Posture (Manual I, ch. 4, p 24)
- While sustaining the Standing Posture simply begin to rhythmically bounce. Stay aware of the softness in your

Mingmen area (low back, sacrum, and tailbone) while you are bouncing. Allow everything else to also stay relaxed.

2. **Bouncing in Side-to-Side Movement** (Manual I, ch. 4, p 35)

3. **Bouncing in Push and Fall** (ch. 2, p 22)
   - For this movement, bring your feet closer together, slightly less than shoulder width.

4. **Bouncing in Tan Tien Turning** (ch. 2, p 20)
   - Bring your feet back out to shoulder width. You must pay extra attention to keeping your Mingmen area soft and relaxed in this movement.

3. Allow the Yin Qi and Yang Qi to Form Their Union of Balance

Qi is the Oneness and Love of God extending itself as vibrational existence. Qi is Creation. Everything in Creation: thoughts, feelings and emotions, and all expressions of energy and matter, is formed from Qi. And the only way that any of these things can exist is because of the balanced giving and receiving naturally and always occurring between the yin and yang forces of Qi. It is this balance that permits the image of God (the reflection of God's infinite beliefs and stories) to appear, to become the infinite vibrational realities of Creation. This is Qi's purpose, Her "gong."

Balance (and integration) is the natural expression of oneness and love within Creation. It is only you and I as extensions of God's Consciousness that can disturb or alter this process of balance. Why we chose and keep on choosing to do this is beyond me, it is the unanswerable question (ch 1, pp 20-21). But what we do, how we continue doing it, and how we can stop doing it are the conversation in "***Experiencing God's Reflection ~ The Role Qi Gong Plays in the Transformation of Consciousness.***"

When you remember that the essence of Who You Are is consciousness, God's Consciousness or Christ Consciousness, you recognize that your identity and value do not come from Qi, or from what you are now experiencing in Her. You know again that you are the Oneness and Love of God. You can then walk forward without attaching your consciousness to the Qi because you no longer feel a need to seek your identity and value in Her. You stop judging, controlling, and manipulating your experiences. You allow the divine intelligence of Creation to form her union of balance within the altars (tan tiens) of your being. In other words, you allow the Qi to do Her gong. These are the actions of the *Essence Movement of Qi Gong Practice* (ch. 13). When you experience life in this way through each of your tan tiens, you are ready for the *Core Event of Qi Gong Practice* (ch. 7).

A. Feel in your movements the rising/expanding/opening expression of Qi (yang), and also feel the sinking/

contracting/closing expression (yin). These two expressions of Qi are simultaneously present in every movement, though in a particular movement you can and may focus your awareness primarily on one expression at a time. Please feel these yang and yin expressions of Qi in the following movements from the Unity Form:

- *Driving Qi Up the Midline, Fingers Leading* (movement 5, p 35)
- *Driving Qi Down the Midline, Elbows Leading* (movement 10, p 38)
- *Driving Qi Up the Midline, Elbows Leading* (movement 3, p 34)
- *Driving Qi Down the Midline, Fingers Leading* (movement 8, p 37)

As you are doing the first movement, can you feel the second movement (its oppositional movement) and visa versa?

As you are doing the third movement, can you feel the forth movement (its oppositional movement) and visa versa?

B. In each movement feel where tension is in your body, and feel the relaxation that is present at the same time. Experience the tension and relaxation expressing in these movements from the "Spinal Series":

1. *Push and Fall* (p 22)
2. *Slow Undulations with Forward and Back Hold* (p 17)

C. Feel the origin of the yang, your push against the earth, and the origin of the yin, all that you internally release. Your push sends energy up through you; your releasing sends energy down through you. In their union, the union of yang and yin, your "peng force" is created.

Chin Circling, a deeper version of the undulations, demonstrates clearly this union of yang and yin as it occurs within your very core (spine and pelvis).

- Stand with your feet slightly wider than shoulder width, keeping your feet parallel. Allow your hands to rest on your hips (where your thigh meets your pelvis).

- While keeping your legs straight and extending through your spine, neck, and head, bend forward as far as you can. At the end of your bending, completely relax your spine, neck, and head, allowing them to hang from your waist. At this point your head is at or below the level of your knees.

- Now slightly bend your knees as you release your low back and pelvis into the sink-fold-release position. At the same time, you must experience a deep and complete relaxation running down through your body from your head to your feet. Also imagine that an energy string lightly connects the top of your head to the tip of your tailbone.

- Not loosing this deep relaxation and the "energy string,"

start to push against the earth in order to rise. This will start your undulation. You will feel a sequential, forward movement come up through your shins, knees, thighs, pelvis, stomach, solar plexus, chest, and neck. During this rising undulation, do not engage your head.

- At the point that your chin starts to lift from your chest, you again straighten your legs and extend through your spine, neck, and head in order to repeat the movement.

D. Now feel how the peng force emanates out from your body (from the five pumps within your body) to fill your energetic field with both expansion and contraction. Experience how your shoulders, arms, and hands release to this force and are moved by it.

A great analogy for this is how a soft silk flag releases itself to the wind that gives it life.

1. In *Whirling Arms* ~ the third movement of the Foundation Form (p 60 in Manual I), experience how your shoulders and arms are carried in the power flowing from the internal pumps of the cua (folding and unfolding of knees and hips), spine (lengthening and shortening of the spine), and chest (opening and closing of the chest).

2. In *Striking with Open Hands* ~ the eighth movement of the Foundation Form (p 69 in Manual I), experience

how the spiral/counter spiral of your spine (fourth internal pump) issues forth and draws in your arms and hands. Also feel how the spiraling in your spine translates into the spiraling/counter spiraling in your arms and hands.

E. Feel the outward reaching and inward drawing flows in your movements. Experience how they are the complementary yang and yin expressions forming the movement.

1. *Cleaning the Rice* ~ second movement of the Unity Form

2. *Scooping Qi from Heaven* ~ seventh movement of the Unity Form

F. Feel where you are giving and where you are receiving. Experience how giving and receiving are the two sides of a single action.

1. *Giving to the Kingdom, Receiving from the Kingdom* ~ sixteenth movement of the Unity Form.

4. Allow Your Body to Unify Physically and Energetically

Every movement begins and is executed in your Lower Tan Tien. The movement then travels to every part of your body through your "peng" and your "silk reeling interconnection". In Internal Arts Practice, this is stated as "when one part moves, all parts move".

Your peng is the energetic field permeating and surrounding your body and, like everything vibrational, comes into existence through the marriage of yin and yang. It is an expression of your etheric Qi. You are able to move in space because of this field, and it is the medium that makes it possible for you to interact and "touch" all things energetic and physical.

All of your movements arise from this field's two expressions: expansion and contraction. You experience your movements of rising, opening, outward reaching, and giving when you intend yang to dominate. You experience your movements of sinking, closing, inward drawing, and receiving when you intend yin to dominate.

In you peng feels like an inner pressure or fullness. It is like the air pressure in a balloon that allows each part of the balloon to be in contact with every other part. When you touch the balloon in one place, you are actually touching all of its other places through its internal pressure ~ through its peng.

Pushing the Wall, Pushing Another
A great way to experience your peng force is to push against a wall or a partner. As you do the following exercise, feel how your peng forms as you allow the yin

force of your relaxed, internal organs to flow downward and through the yang force that is naturally flowing up through you when you push.

- Find a sturdy wall. With feet together, face the wall at slightly more than arms length distance, then drop your arms to your sides.

- To push against the wall, you will need to be in a Bow Stance. So pivot your right foot so the toes point 45° to the right. Slightly bend your knee as you place all of your weight into your right leg. Then extend your left foot forward and approximately three inches to the left with the toes pointing directly at the wall. Your toes need to be about 8–10 inches from the wall.

- Turn so that your pelvis, chest, and head face the wall. Check to see that you have the three-inch cannel running between your feet from front to back.

- Form the Standing Posture, remembering the six adjustments, the relaxation of your internal organs (and pelvic floor), and reciprocal extension through your spine. The tip of your tongue touches the roof of your mouth.

- Now place your open hands on the wall, fingers pointing up, shoulder width apart, and at chest height.

- Remember how to connect your arms to your body. With your hands flat on the wall, really feel the downward heaviness in your shoulders and elbows; your elbows must be unlocked and your elbow tips must be pointing down. At the same time, feel an internal extending or lengthening through your shoulders, arms, and hands.

- Start by pushing very lightly against the wall. Feel the energy bridge forming through your body from your back foot, through your sacrum (the key stone), to your open palms. STAY AWARE OF THIS ENERGY LINE WHEN YOU INCREASE THE POWER OF YOUR PUSH!

- Begin slowly to push more and more from your back foot. But for each ounce of increased pushing (the yang force, which will naturally flow up through your body, through the energy line, to your palms and to the top of your head) you must allow an equal amount of relaxation (the yin force) to flow downward.

- The resulting feeling of an expansion or fullness, permeating and surrounding your body, is your peng.

Peng With a Partner
- You can enhance your experience of peng, your peng and their peng, with a partner. Start by facing one another at slightly more than arms length, which is with both of you extending your arms. You both then drop your arms.

- Both of you now pivot your right foot 45°, and both extend your left foot toward your partner. Each of you must have a three-inch channel and the tips of your toes sit even with and approximately five inches to the side of your partner's.

- Turn your pelvis, chest, and head to face one another. Each of you places your left, open palm on the center of your partner's chest, fingers pointing up. Your right hands cup your partner's left elbow.

- Form your Standing Posture.

- Then proceed as if you were pushing against the wall... Start slowly, first feeling the energy bridge forming through your body (from your back foot, through your sacrum, to the palm you have placed on their chest). Then, as you begin to push more, allow the relaxation within your body to flow down in proportion to the strength of the push coming up through you from your back foot.

Contracting Peng

When working with a partner, you can also experience the contracting expression of your peng.

- Change your hand positions. With your left, grab your partner's left or right arm (does not matter which) just above the elbow; with your right, grab their wrist.

- You will now be pulling your partner, so begin slowly by lightly pushing from your front, left foot.

- Make sure that you are still in the Standing Posture. Feel the energy line, the bridge forming through your body from your front foot, through your sacrum, to both of your hands.

- Just as before, you must allow the relaxation within your body to flow down in proportion to the increasing strength of the push coming up through you from your front foot.

- The resulting feeling of a contracting, drawing in, and shrinking, permeating and surrounding your body, is your peng. PAY SPECIAL ATTENTION TO THE DEEP, DOWNWARD DRAW IN YOUR SACRUM!

Silk Reeling Interconnection

Your silk reeling interconnection is how the spiraling expression of Qi moves through your body. This understanding takes its name from the way a thread of silk (or any fiber for that matter) is made from the twisting together of many individual fibers. The phenomena is clearly demonstrated when a person holding one end of a rope twists it, and the person holding the other end then experiences that twisting. The silk reeling is how that energy travels through the rope.

The Qi expressions of "peng" and "silk reeling interconnection" are interrelated; they are parts of each other. Peng helps silk reeling and silk reeling helps peng. If the rope is held taut, the twisting force can travel more quickly and powerfully through the rope.

Distributing and Balancing the Qi, the eighteenth movement of the Unity Form (p 44), is an excellent example of how the spiraling in your spine (pump 4) travels throughout your body ~ from your feet to the tips of your fingers.

In *Circling the Tan Tien*, watch how the circling within my lower abdomen, which I am tracing with my hands, becomes a circling in my chest, and then becomes the way I am moving my head.

In *Hand Circling*, watch how the same lower abdominal circle not only becomes the circling in my chest, but now travels through my shoulder, elbow, and wrist, to finally express as a circling in my hand and fingers.

5. Express Greatly from Your Heart

Remember, you are the Consciousness of Oneness and Love, the Christ Consciousness forever present within your Spiritual Heart. Through the extraordinary relationship your heart has with your Spiritual Body (ch. 9, pp 129, 130), you, even now, are consciously experiencing your Soul and the oneness and love you share with God, Creation and all life.

Your mind, the Upper Tan Tien, is your sky mirror. In its highest function it is giving you a mental reflection of the oneness and love existing within your Spiritual Heart. Your body, the Lower Tan Tien, is your earth mirror. In its highest function it is giving you an energetic and physical reflection of this same truth forever present within this deepest heart.

- In your practice allow your heart, even in its physical movement, to openly and greatly express.

  1. In *Offering Your Heart* (Unity Form movement 15, p 41), allow your heart to hugely open and close; let it reach out infinitely and gather in infinitely.

  2. In *Spiral Open, Spiral Close* (Foundation Form movement 6, Manual I, p 65), allow your heart to not only open and close, but powerfully express your spiraling to the left and right.

6. Use "Imaginative Feeling" to allow the Functions of your Tan Tiens to Integrate

In the theory of Qi Gong you are oneness. In the practice of Qi Gong you consciously experience this oneness by allowing what you have perceived to be the pieces and levels of yourself to return into a unified whole (ch. 8, pp 104-106).

Right now you are choosing to believe that you are formed from separate pieces: a Soul, consciousness, mind, heart, and body, and that you exist separate from God, Creation, and your brothers and sisters. You also are choosing to be limited in your power.... in your power to love, manifest your will, and commune with Creation and all life.

These are the beliefs that you are now bringing before the mirror of Creation. And in Her infinite power, Creation is reflecting these beliefs to you perfectly as your experiences. These reflections are your present reality.

As you walk the Qi Gong path, you realize oneness by allowing a reintegration to occur within you. Through this process, you again know that the Oneness, Love, and Unlimited Power of God are you, you remember Who You Are, and therefore experience this in the world surrounding you as well.

Integration occurs naturally within you when you move with "Imaginative Feeling" - YOU DEEPLY <u>FEEL</u> <u>MEANING</u> IN <u>DOING</u>.

- When doing your practice, "see" your movements (visualization), understand and give meaning to them, through your Upper Tan Tien.

- Through your Middle Tan Tien feel your movements.

- And, of course, physically execute your movements through your Lower Tan Tien.

- Use your Imaginative Feeling to integrate all of these functions.

The deep art of moving through "Imaginative Feeling" is clearly palpable in the following movements:

1. *Grabbing the Tree's Qi* (Foundation Form movement 9, Manual I, p 72).

    - When spiraling the tan tiens to face forward, lengthening your spine and opening your chest, and allowing your arms and hands to flow up and out, deeply feel your energetic field expanding out to encompass the beauty in front of you.

    - Then, when your tan tiens spiral back to the diagonal, your spine is shortening and chest closing, and you are grabbing and drawing your arms down and in, deeply feel your energetic field contracting, and how it is pulling and receiving into you all of this beauty.

2. *Close* (Foundation Form last movement, Manual I, p 76.).

    - With your first rise and the opening out of your wings become present in and feel your heart.

    - As you sink and then draw up with long fingers, connect deeply with the earth, your Mother. Bring Her into your heart, allow Her Qi to become your Qi.

- As you abruptly sink and then slowly rise, allow your Qi to then enter the base of your spine in order to flow up your back to the top of your head.

- Through your slight sink/rise, allow the power of your sink to carry your arms out to heaven and the power of your rise to draw heaven's Qi into your head, to also become your Qi.

- Now, in your final sink and then rise, allow your Qi to flow down the front of your body to your heart (Middle Tan Tien), and then continue down to your lower abdomen (Lower Tan Tien). Deeply feel how the blending of Earth and Heaven within your internal orbit (the Microcosmic Orbit) unifys you with all existence!

7. What Happens in One Tan Tien Happens in all Tan Tiens

This understanding speaks clearly to the overarching spirituality of Qi Gong Practice. It does not matter through which tan tien you initiate your practice or are experiencing, for what you allow or facilitate on any one level of your being simultaneously occurs on all the other levels.

When you allow the yin and yang expressions of Qi to flow into one another in a physical movement, you are allowing this union of balance to occur in the astral and causal levels. And when you choose to not attach your consciousness (your identity and personal value) to either the yin side or the yang side of an emotional or mental experience, you are also allowing the Qi to form her union of balance in the other tan tiens.

This principle holds true with each and every experience you have on every level of your existence.

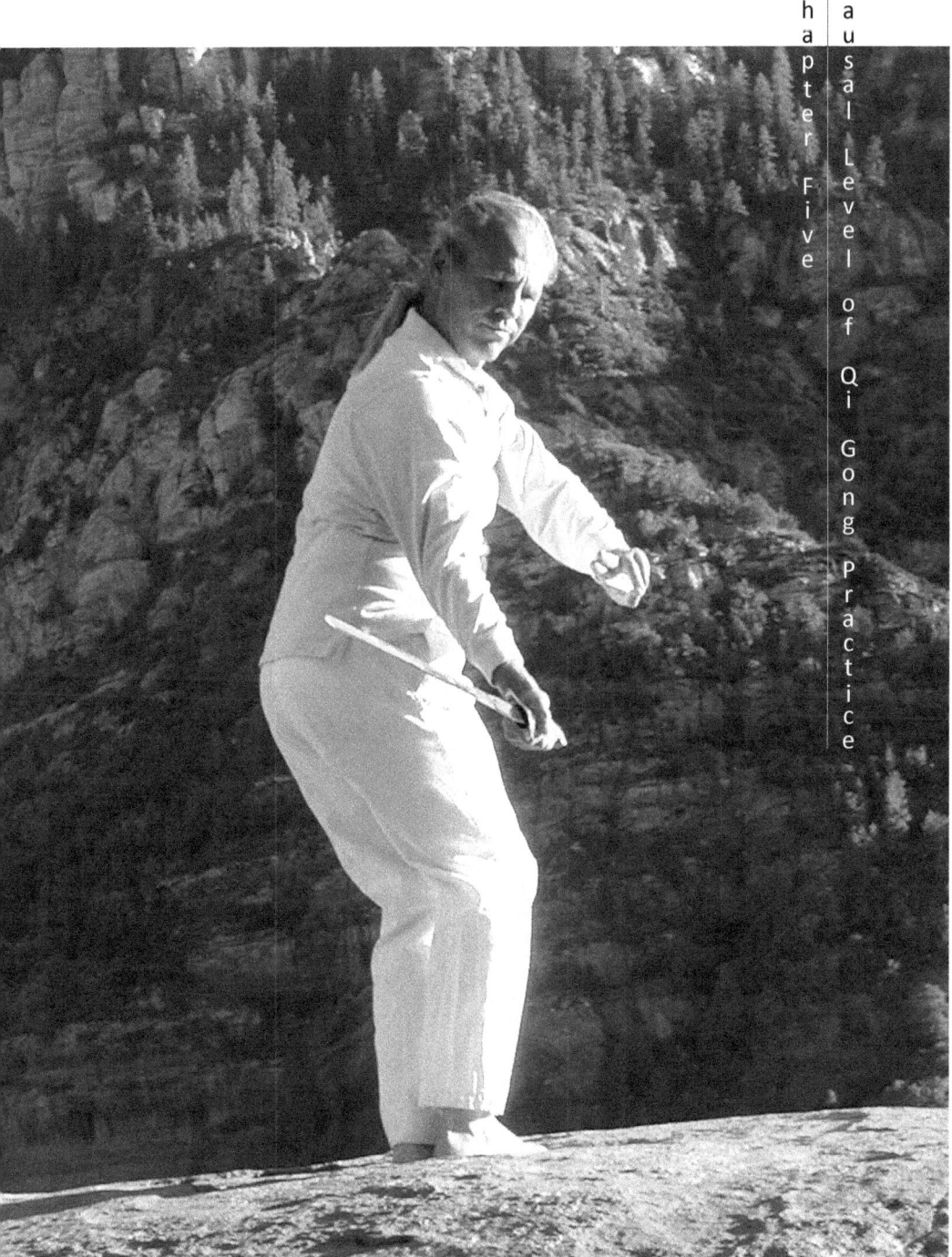

Chapter Five — Causal Level of Qi Gong Practice

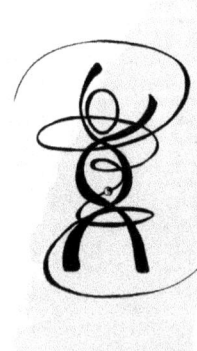

Meditation of Three Levels

PREPARE TO MEDITATE BY SITTING on a cushion or safu that elevates your pelvis 2-3 inches, and cross your legs. Another option is to sit on the edge of a firm, flat chair with your legs extended forward and slightly to the sides, just enough so that your knees are slightly below the level of your hips.

Place your left hand on top of the right, palms up, thumb tips lightly touching. Your hands rest comfortably on your lap; your shoulders, arms, and hands are completely relaxed (if you hands fall apart, it is not a problem).

First Level

This meditation practice starts in your foundation, the physical/energetic or Etheric level of your being. Starting here gives you a very real, tangible entrance to the inner path.

The balance you allow between the yin and yang Qi of this level sets a powerful precedent that facilitates the balance between these forces in the other levels in which you exist and experience... the Astral and Causal.

Create a preliminary alignment through you body.
- Lightly pull up on a string that attaches at the Bai Hui point (this point is where a line connecting the tops of your ears would pass over the top of your head).

- While still pulling up on this "string", bring your chin slightly down and slightly towards you (the tip of your chin moves a little towards your Adam's apple).

- Then slightly bend at your hips in order to incline your spine a few degrees forward.

Feel the yin force
- Take your awareness within you and completely relax all of your internal organs: brain, lungs and heart, liver, stomach, spleen, intestines, and kidneys.

- Allow the heaviness of theses relaxed organs to pass down through your body as if it were silt settling to the bottom of a pond. It is okay if your lower back slightly slumps at this juncture.

- Really feel the weight of your relaxed organs pressing down into the cushion or chair.

<u>Feel the yang force</u>

- Now imagine this heaviness to be the rich mud that has formed at the bottom of your pond. This heavy, rich mud is the energy that feeds the lotus plant of your spine. Out of this heaviness, your spine now grows upward through you, to the top of your head. At this point, your spine literally lengthens as it is reaching for heaven. Your low back is now no longer slumped.

- Once this internal dynamic is established in you and you are confident with it, it is time to relax your outer, muscular body as well. Allow the heaviness of your relaxed, outer body to also pass downward in order to further feed the yang forces moving upward through your spine.

Take care at this juncture, for even though the spine is lengthening as it grows towards heaven, it cannot up root itself from the mud. You must sustain both sensations in your body simultaneously – the heavy mud of your relaxed body, and the upward, growing lotus of your spine. <u>The key is to "feel" that the heaviness of your relaxation is causing the lengthening of your spine</u>.

- The balance of these two forces is the portal into your etheric body. This body of energy extends into infinity, and your experience of being in this body is like floating or being suspended. For approximately five minutes (longer if you wish), allow yourself to expand outwardly as far as you are comfortable. Sense how everything that is happening around you is taking place within the great stillness of your infinite, etheric body.

- To close this level of the meditation, simply bring your attention back inside of your lower abdomen, just below your navel.

Second Level

This level of the meditation is about feeling... feeling the flow of Qi as it is moving freely and effortlessly through the altars or tan tiens of your temple. Here you experience that the feeling function of your Astral Altar is the key to unifying yourself. This effortless flow of Qi through the Middle Tan Tien opens your heart to encompass all the pieces and levels of your being.

This reunification of your being forms your Spiritual Body and opens the mystical way to consciously experience the pure reflection of your Soul. This is the Core Event of Qi Gong Practice (ch. 7), your conscious experience of being the oneness and love unifying God, all Creation, and all consciousness.

- Recheck your posture. Are you still in the "floating feeling" arising from the marriage of the yin (heavy release) and the yang (upward growing) Qi of your etheric body? If not, re-establish this state.

- With your awareness, walk from your Qi Hai point (two inches below your navel) inward toward your spine. In this place, envision your central channel (the Chong

Meridian). This channel, much like an elevator shaft running in front of the spine, channels the Qi from the Lower Tan Tien (the etheric field in your lower abdomen and pelvis) through the Middle Tan Tien (the astral field in the center of your chest) to the Upper Tan Tien (the causal field in the center of your brain).

- Enter into this channel. On your inhale feel your awareness flow upward through this channel, passing effortlessly through the heart space into the center of your brain. On your exhale feel your awareness flow downward, passing effortlessly through the heart space, into your lower abdomen and pelvis. Allow the Qi to run through this channel for approximately three minutes (longer if you wish).

Again, take care at this juncture. It is not your breath that is moving through this channel. It is your awareness or "your sense of self." This movement is, therefore, effortless!

- If you have trouble feeling your tan tiens, a powerful tool is to – on the first run, pause within each tan tien and experience, through your "imaginative feeling", the sound "I'm" emanating from that tan tien three times. Do this within all three tan tiens on the way up, and then experience this sound just once in the Middle Tan Tien, and Lower Tan Tien on the way down. Then you can proceed with the meditation, simply allowing the Qi to flow effortlessly up and down through the central channel and the three tan tiens.

- Finish this level of the meditation by having your awareness stay within the Upper Tan Tien, the center point of your brain.

Third Level

<u>The third level of the meditation is a powerful and key part in the causal practice of Qi Gong</u>. Our ego or "I Am" consciousness (the consciousness of conscious experience (ch. 3, pp 39-41), has identified itself with our Causal Altar or Tan Tien (ch. 10, pp 155-157). We have quite literally come to believe that we are our thoughts, and that this "thinking self" that we believe we are is superior to our heart and body and all the other aspects of Creation. Our mind has become the home of our ego, our belief in a separate self and a separated existence. It has become "our new god."

Through this level of the meditation, we observe the continuous dance between the comparative or complementary expressions of causal Qi (ch. 15, pp 227, 228). We experience that our consciousness does not come from this interplay of meanings, and we come to know again that these thoughts are not Who We Are.

- Recheck your posture. Are you in the "floating feeling?" If not, re-establish this state.

- So there you are, sitting within the center of your own brain. How you allow the causal Qi to form her union of balance, and how you experience this balance through this altar, is a bit different:

- BE AWARE OF ABSOLUTELY EVERYTHING, EVERYTHING THAT SURROUNDS YOU, AND ALL OF THE THOUGHTS AND FEELINGS WITHIN YOU.
- BUT CHOOSE NO ONE THING. ALLOW YOUR AWARENESS TO TOUCH EACH THING EQUALLY.

This experience is much like watching a river flow by. Every now and then something does catch your eye, but you choose to let it go as your awareness returns to "watching" the whole river.

- Hold this state of omnipresence for approximately five minutes (longer if you wish).

If a thought or feeling, or a sensory input from the world around you becomes "sticky", in that it attracts or holds your awareness repetitively, gently apply these two helpers:

— Say to yourself:
"I release, I'm not this thought or feeling, I am love. I'm not the future or the past, I am this moment."

— Then re-form your posture: Pull on your string, adjust your chin, and slightly incline your spine forward. Allow your inner and outer bodies to relax, feeling how their heaviness feeds your lengthening spine. The tip of your tongue touches the roof of your mouth.

Then proceed with the meditation... BE AWARE OF EVERYTHING, BUT CHOOSE NO ONE THING. ALLOW YOUR AWARENESS TO TOUCH EACH THING EQUALLY.

- To close the meditation, bring your awareness back into your Lower Tan Tien, two inches below your navel. When you are fully present within yourself and in the present moment, simply open your eyes.

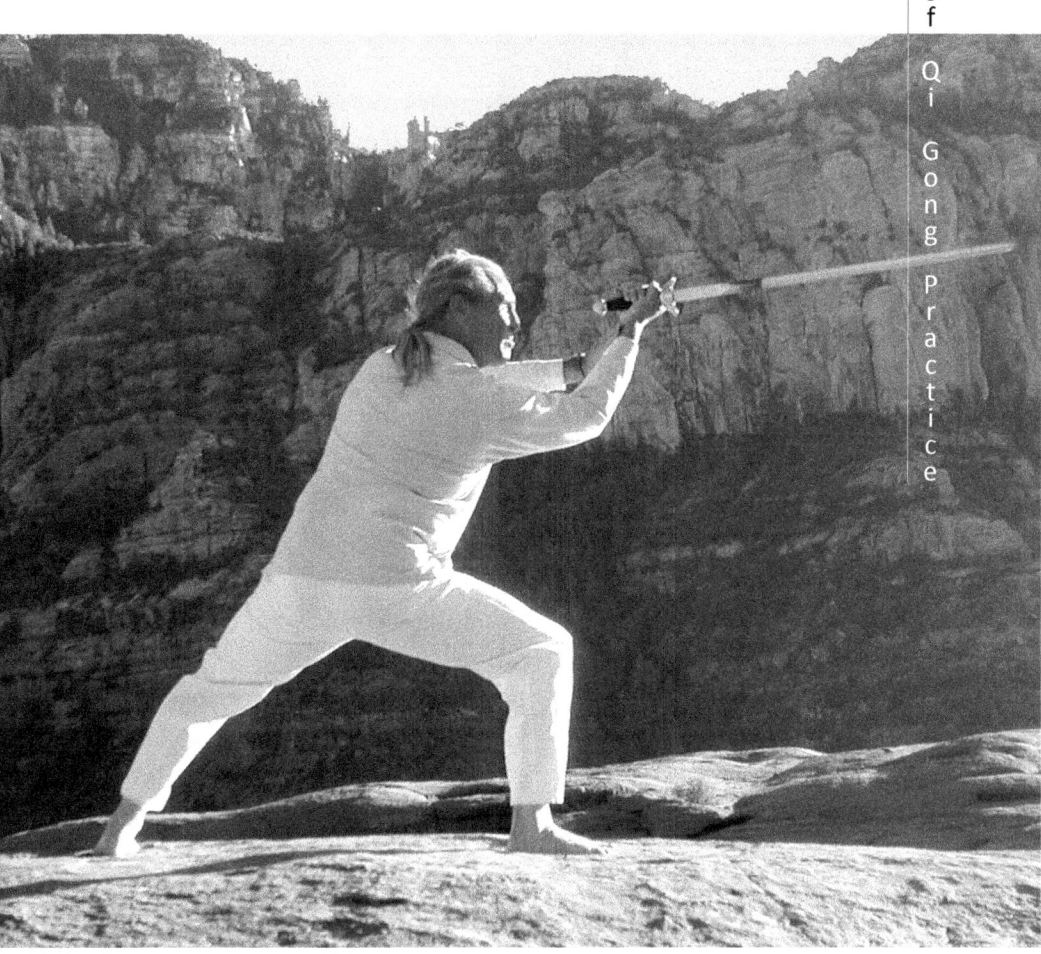

Chapter Six: Astral Level of Qi Gong Practice

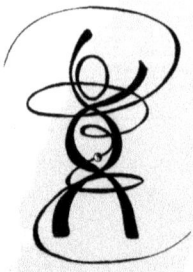

The Astral Practice of Qi Gong

It is your everyday life that gives you the greatest opportunities to practice astral Qi Gong. Especially in this present timing, all of us are experiencing strong feelings and emotions regarding Who We Are, and what our role is in every arena of our life – personal relationships, health, work, finances, politics, environmental concerns, and spirituality.

Your feelings and emotions are your experiences of the astral Qi of Creation, which come to your consciousness through your Astral Altar or Middle Tan Tien. Just like with your thoughts (causal Qi) and perceptions of energy and matter (etheric Qi), you experience each feeling and emotion (astral Qi) as having two opposing sides, a yin side and a yang side (ch. 15 p 229).

The root of why you experience absolutely everything in

your reality (thoughts, emotions, and physical/energetic things) as a duality is because you believe that there exists a power opposing God. In your forgetting that there is only God (Oneness), and in the confusion brought on by your experiences of the reflections in Creation of such an untruth, you have gone on to believe that:

— your identity and value come from Qi and what you are experiencing in Her,

— you are divided within yourself and exist separate from God and Creation,

— and you are limited in your power to love, manifest your will, and commune with Creation.

Furthermore, you continue, without even knowing it, to bind your consciousness to experiencing all these untruths through your judgments and acts of control and manipulation (ch. 5, p 63 and ch. 10, pp 156-158, 163-165).

In the astral practice of Qi Gong, you become aware of the dual nature of each of your emotions. You also see how you, by judging and identifying with your emotional experiences, have hidden deep within your being (in your subconscious and semi conscious self) aspects of your emotions that have hurt you, and you have felt you cannot live with. In doing this, you literally divide an emotion into yin and yang halves. Deep within yourself you then incarcerate one half, the hurtful half, of this emotion, keeping it apart from its corresponding partner. This process requires tremendous amounts of energy to maintain and only drains you and obscures your truth.

The primary intention in all levels of Qi Gong Practice is to remember Who You Are, to remember that you are oneness and love. In the astral practice, you are reminded that your identity and value do not come from the experiences of your emotions, and therefore you need not judge them. When you cease to judge and no longer feel the need to control and manipulate the astral Qi and the reflections within her, you allow the yin and yang halves of your emotions to find one another. You are trusting and allowing the intelligence of the Qi (Creation or God Our Mother) to form Her union of balance.

Remember, the balance between the yin and yang forces of Qi, the balance She is always creating, forms the mirror in which you experience God and your own, true self. It is only you, your consciousness, through unnatural attachment and judgment that interferes in this natural process.

The key is:
DO NOT REACT – DO NOT REPRESS

Absolutely everything in Creation is formed from Qi, everything is vibrating, including your emotions. Also at work throughout Creation is the law of harmonics – how something vibrating at a certain frequency can resonate or connect with something else. It is through this phenomenon that your everyday life becomes your teacher in the practice of astral Qi Gong.

Here is how it works. You are walking along the path of your life when something occurs. This occurrence just happens to be vibrating at a frequency that connects to one of the emotions you have incarcerated deep within your being. Having been stimulated through this connection, this aspect of emotion, this half of an emotion that you have judged to be hurtful and intolerable, is released to come into your conscious mind. In your conscious mind, this half of your emotion is now free to find its other half, its natural partner. But, of course, you as consciousness, now get to feel again this aspect of your emotion, an emotion that you not only judged in your past to be hurtful and intolerable, but that you also attached your identity and value to enough to feel you had to hide it. In this experience, life now gives you an opportunity to unbind your consciousness from this emotion and from this limited reality of separation. All you have to do is truly experience this emotion, choosing this time to not react to it (to not use this emotion as your motive for action) and not repress it (to, through your remembrance that your identity and value do not come from this experience, not judge this emotion and not hide any part of it within yourself).

Through your courage to feel your emotions and your choice to not react or repress them, you begin to experience your emotions in a "new way". In this way, you also allow the tremendous energy required to keep these "good" and "bad" halves apart, to reintegrate into your being.

Without your interference, the astral Qi is again free to do Her gong; She can again be the mirror that reflects to you the pure image of God and your Soul. The wholeness of your emotions then serves you, reminding you of your oneness.

In the book, the main references to the astral practice of Qi Gong are in chapter 8, pp 107-108, chapter 9, pp 136-143 and chapter 15, pp 229-230.

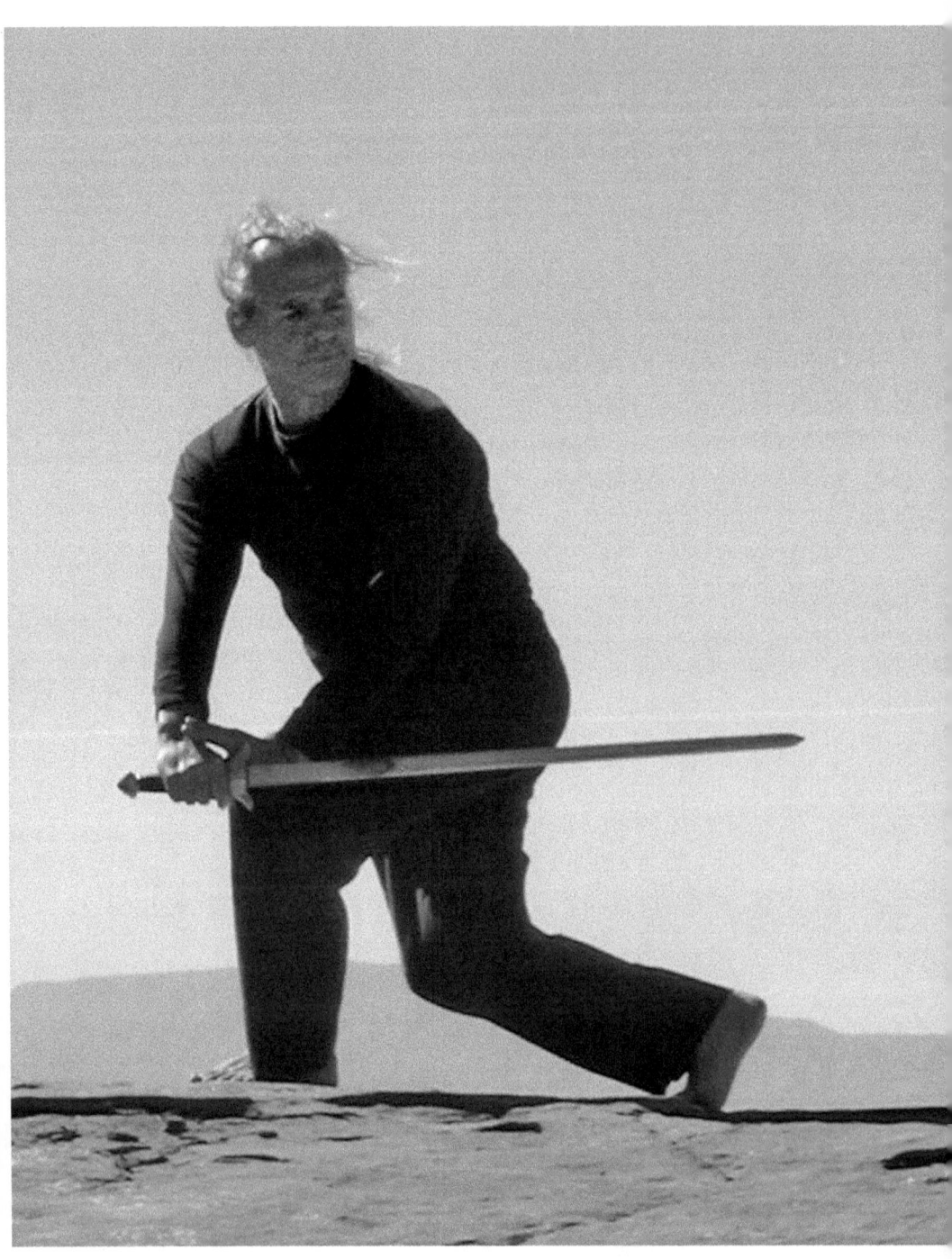

About the Author

Lyn Dilbeck is a thirty-year practitioner of Qi Gong and Internal Martial Arts. He currently lives in Sedona, Arizona where he has been teaching these arts for the past twenty years.

To know himself and to help others know themselves has always been the deepest motivating force in Lyn's life. This heart-felt desire is the essence of his Qi Gong Practice and what he shares as a teacher.

Before Lyn started to develop a conscious relationship with Qi through Qi Gong Practice, his quest had taken him into metaphysics and the practice of meditation. Also having a desire to help others, he studied and practiced medicine as a Pediatric and Internal Medicine Physicians Assistant. These earlier studies and life experiences helped him to see that the power and intelligence that give us health is what heals us when we are ill. He felt that this intelligent power must be what sustains every level of our existence ~ physical, energetic, emotional and mental, and it must be connected somehow to the life purpose within each of us.

For Lyn, accepting that health, healing and spirituality were interconnected, was an epiphany that changed the direction of his life. He decided to seek out this intelligent power, to know it within himself, and to help others to know it within themselves.

In the mid-seventies, many people seeking a physical/energetic practice based in spirituality were studying Yoga, Aikido or Tai Qi Chuan. Lyn studied all three forms, yet it was in the practice of the traditional Yang Style of Tai Qi Chuan that he experienced those first "tastes" of a force flowing in and around him.

Lyn has come to know Qi Gong Practice as a conscious conversation between human beings and the intelligent power of Creation, Qi. In the course of this conversation he has learned that Qi is the divine intelligence and power that is birthing God's infinite potential into Creation. This is her true gong (purpose), to be the Mother of all vibrational existence and our Mother as well.

Lyn has spent the majority of his life tending this relationship and been fortunate to study with many gifted masters of Qi Gong and Internal Martial Arts:
- Ralf Cahn, Albany, CA ~ Kang jo fu
- Stephen Labensart, Mt. Shasta, CA ~ Yang Style Tai Qi Chuan
- Lily Soux, Honolulu, HI ~ Qi Gong
- George Xu, San Francisco, CA ~ Chen Style Tai Qi Chuan

- Chris Luth, Solano Beach, CA ~ Push Hands Training
- Master Zhou Ting Jue, Los Angeles, CA ~ Qi Gong (Wu Dang Style), Tai Qi Chuan, Hsing I, Bagua
- Miranda Warburton, Flagstaff, AZ ~ Hsing I, Bagua
- Master Li Jun Feng, Austin, TX ~ Sheng Zhen Qi Gong
- Master Chris Petrilli, Sedona, AZ ~ Escrima

Passionate and generous in all that he shares; Lyn excels in revealing the internal principles of these arts through demonstration and metaphor. His deeper gift however, is the way he shows that these principles are the same keys that allow our true nature to manifest into our life as joy, wisdom, health and love.

In addition to his own practice and teaching, Lyn is a lover of nature. You can often find him on a lake or river, boating and camping. He loves Mexico where he has lived and traveled; he also teaches Spanish as a second language.

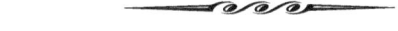

FOR MORE INFORMATION about these teachings, Lyn's workshops, or hosting a workshop in your area, please contact Lyn via his website: www.spiralinglifeforce.com

www.ingramcontent.com/pod-product-compliance
Lightning Source LLC
Chambersburg PA
CBHW071737090426
42738CB00011B/2508